D1614733

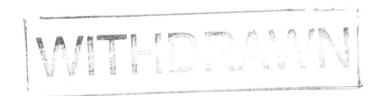

Public Health Intelligence

Krishna Regmi • Ivan Gee
Editors

Public Health Intelligence

Issues of Measure and Method

Foreword by Prof. Mala Rao and David Kidney

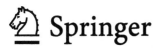 Springer

Editors
Krishna Regmi
University of Bedfordshire
Luton, United Kingdom

Ivan Gee
Liverpool John Moores University
Liverpool, United Kingdom

ISBN 978-3-319-28324-1   ISBN 978-3-319-28326-5   (eBook)
DOI 10.1007/978-3-319-28326-5

Library of Congress Control Number: 2016933317

Printed on acid-free paper

This Springer imprint is published by Springer Nature
The registered company is Springer International Publishing AG Switzerland

Foreword

During the past three decades, epidemiology, the study of the distribution and determinants of health and disease and the application of this knowledge to the prevention and control of disease and to healthcare, has made great strides. In large part this is due to the development of information technology and access to new knowledge. In parallel, the evidence-based healthcare movement evolved, replacing conventional wisdom, opinion and tradition which were often the basis for healthcare choices with decisions based on the findings of rigorous scientific research.

In the wider public arena, the previous tendency was for political, social and economic discourse about health to revolve narrowly around healthcare services or even more narrowly around acute hospital care provision. Thankfully, this has gradually given way to an increasing recognition of the crucial impact of socioeconomic and other environmental determinants on population health and wellbeing. There is a much sharper focus now on the need to address these wider determinants of health and wellbeing at population levels: going upstream to maximise the prevention opportunities. And although values, vested interests and political opinion continue to play a significant role in influencing health decisions, increasingly, high-quality research-derived information as well as the growing demand for public accountability and transparency are driving a more evidence-based public health policy development, planning and implementation. In the global arena too, population health is undergoing a major epidemiological shift in response to a landscape of rapid social, economic and environmental change. Health and social inequalities are widening, and the past predominance of communicable diseases is being replaced by an increasing prevalence of non-communicable diseases. Evidence-based approaches to address these challenges and achieve health equity will inevitably require systematic collection, synthesis and review of data from multiple sources reflecting the wider determinants of disease, a big task and one that will only be successfully undertaken with the 'right skills at the right place and at the right time'.

And this, of course, is where the role of public health intelligence comes in. Our enthusiasm for this text comes with a particular interest. Our backgrounds of having led the development of the UK Public Health Skills and Career Framework, now known as the Public Health Skills and Knowledge Framework (MR), and as the executive director of the Public Health Register (DK) explain our concern that strengthening workforce knowledge and capability to improve public health nationally and globally remains a priority.

The Framework, which set out for the first time in the UK and possibly worldwide the competencies and underpinning knowledge base required across the public health delivery system, established surveillance and assessment of population health needs as core competencies required of the whole public health delivery system and public health intelligence as a defined area of specialisation. And the groundbreaking Public Health Register, the first independent regulator for multidisciplinary public health professionals not covered by another regulatory body, included public health intelligence professionals within its ambit. These two developments confirmed the central importance of public health information and intelligence capability in systems aimed at improving population health and wellbeing. More recently, further recognition of the need for high calibre information and intelligence expertise at all levels of the system has come from the development of guidance by the Faculty of Public Health to establish a common approach for the recruitment of public health information and intelligence staff across different organisations, as well as a 2014 Faculty of Public Health report reaffirming public health intelligence as a key function required to be delivered by a local public health system.

Against this background the ill-defined training pathways for these staff have been a concern. A lack of authoritative textbooks to underpin the training in this specialised area of public health practice has been another significant obstacle, in terms of resources to facilitate the enhancement of appropriate knowledge and skills, until now, that is, when this glaring gap has been addressed by the publication of this book which is set to become a 'must-read' not only for those intending to specialise in health intelligence but for the entire public health workforce. In this book, probably the first of its kind, the professional analysis, interpretation and presentation of population information in support of health and wellbeing decision-making at every level of society is expertly explained and explored. Made up of 12 chapters, the book takes the reader systematically from the historical context to a fascinating picture of a future landscape a decade from now in which changes in digital technology are predicted to be slowing down and the focus is increasingly on the human–technology interface.

Public health practice in the UK is described as being made up of three domains, health services, health protection and health improvement, and three underpinning functions which include public health intelligence. This book amply demonstrates why public health intelligence is simply indispensable to the process of making informed decisions based on appropriate and reliable evidence.

And whose decisions should be so informed? Why, everyone's!

Health needs to be at the heart of all the politicians' and other policymakers' decisions and at the heart of every individual's decisions that will impact on their own health and wellbeing as well as the health and wellbeing of their families and their communities.

We very much hope that as well as establishing the centrality of public health intelligence to good decision-making in our society, this book will demonstrate the need to recognise and respect the work of the people who strive to provide us with this information in the first place.

They are such a valuable public health resource, the men and women who gather, analyse, interpret and communicate evidence. They are our guides and teachers in matters of epidemiology, surveillance, research methods and synthesis of the information related to health and wellbeing.

We must invest appropriately in their education and training and their continuing development. When you read this book, you will appreciate the skills and knowledge needed in terms of management and communication of knowledge. It clearly demonstrates the importance of equipping this workforce with the ability to support all of us so that we live our lives in the best possible health.

Imperial College London & formerly, Head of Public Health   Mala Rao
Workforce and Capacity, Department of Health for England, UK

UK Public Health Register, Birmingham, UK   David Kidney

Preface

Public health systems worldwide have recognised the importance of basing local action on evidence and local intelligence, and appropriate decision-making in healthcare practice requires reliable health intelligence. Our academic and professional experience—nationally and globally—show that due to several challenges faced in the emerging public health paradigm, traditional research may no longer be appropriate for addressing complex public health interventions, and the systems that are required should ensure that public health professionals can access the right knowledge at the right time. We, therefore, believe that providing and utilising appropriate health intelligence (information, data, knowledge, evidence and analysis) by policy planners and decision-makers at local levels will allow the best decisions to be made and will ultimately bring lasting change in people's health and wellbeing status (WHO 2014).

Health intelligence now has clearly defined career ladders in the health sector, ranging from the positions of practitioners to specialists or even consultants; at the time of writing this preface, there are no existing academic texts that would facilitate appropriate transfer of knowledge, skills and aptitude through education and training. It is felt that there is a real need for a textbook on public health intelligence and how evidence and intelligence are used to inform policy at a local, national and international level.

The two distinguishing features of the book are:

- This book will provide some critical understanding of the principles, analytical techniques, toolkits and methods in health intelligence.
- This book will be the first academic text on public health intelligence and will be a significant contribution to translating evidence into policy in the public health community.

Primarily, this book should be essential reading for those involved in public health healthcare, including allied healthcare students, graduate professionals or practitioners, providing them with the opportunity to become confident users of public health evidence.

The book is structured in ways that introduce the topic to students and practitioners and that provide practical examples or discussion tasks of how different forms of evidence have been used in public health or healthcare sciences and to what ends they would be useful. Each chapter will:

- Define the theme in an accessible way
- Illustrate its application and significance in the field
- Identify and explore issues surrounding the theme
- Provide several references for recommended reading

To make readers more informed and interactive, throughout the book we have employed various 'learner-centred' approaches, for example, 'discussion tasks' and 'case studies', as individual and group activities, in the hope that this will provide readers with some idea of what it is and how it should be discussed/carried out. Any remaining errors are, of course, our own.

Luton, UK   Krishna Regmi
Liverpool, UK   Ivan Gee

Reference

World Health Organisation (2014). *Providing health intelligence to meet local needs: A practical guide to serving local and urban communities through public health observatories*. Geneva, Switzerland: WHO

Acknowledgements

Writing a book as comprehensive as *Public Health Intelligence: Issues of Measure and Method* is not an easy job. We have, however, received wonderful guidance and support from the wider academics and professionals who have made our writing journey a bit less stressful. We would like to thank all the contributors who authored their chapters, spending much time on producing good quality chapters. In addition, we would also like to thank Dr. Alison Hill, Public Health England; Dr. Ananda Allan, Public Health, NHS Dumfries and Galloway, UK; Professor Gurch Randhawa, University of Bedfordshire, UK; Dr. Colin Thunhurst, Coventry University, UK; David Kidney, UK Public Health Register; Dr. Fiona Sim, Royal Society of Public Health, UK; Professor Kristen Kurland, Carnegie Mellon University, USA; Professor Mala Rao, Imperial College London and former Department of Health England; Margaret Eames, London Borough of Newham, UK; Neil Bendel, Public Health Manchester, UK; Dr. Paul Pilkington, University of the West of England, Bristol; and Rose Khatri, Liverpool John Moores University, UK, for sharing their ideas and suggestions while preparing this book. Finally, we appreciate Janet Kim, Khristine Queja and Christina Tuballes, Springer Publications, and the publication team for guiding us to organise the final chapters in a publishable and presentable format!

K. Regmi and I. Gee, *United Kingdom, 2015*

Contents

The Future Directions of Health Intelligence.. 225
  Alison Hill and Julian Flowers

Contributors

Neil Bendel Public Health, Manchester City Council, Manchester, UK

Isabelle Bray Department of Health and Social Sciences, Faculty of Health and Applied Sciences, University of the West of England, Bristol, UK

Adam Briggs Nuffield Department of Population Health, University of Oxford, Oxford, UK

Susan J. Cliffe Independant Consultant, St Albans, UK

Jacqui Dorman Public Health, Tameside MBC, Oldham, UK

Julian Flowers Knowledge and Intelligence Service, Public Health England, Cambridge, UK

Ivan Gee Center for Public Health, Liverpool John Moores University, Liverpool, UK

Ruth Gilbert Faculty of Health and Social Sciences, University of Bedfordshire, Luton, UK

Alison Hill Better Value Healthcare Ltd., Oxford, UK

Katie Johnson Norfolk and Norwich University Hospitals NHS Foundation Trust (on behalf of Health Education East of England), Norwich, UK

Kristen Kurland H. John Heinz III College and School of Architecture, Carnegie Mellon University, Pittsburgh, PA, USA

Krishna Regmi Faculty of Health and Social Sciences, University of Bedfordshire, Luton, UK

Peter Scarborough Nuffield Department of Population Health, University of Oxford, Oxford, UK

Adrian Smith Nuffield Department of Population Health, University of Oxford, Oxford, UK

Colin Thunhurst Faculty of Health and Life Sciences, Coventry University, Coventry, UK

Patrick Tobi Institute for Health and Human Development, University of East London, Stratford, UK

About the Contributors

Neil Bendel, B.A. (Hons.), M.Sc. is a public health specialist with responsibility for public health intelligence at Manchester City Council. He has more than 20 years of experience in public health and public health intelligence in both NHS and local government settings at regional and district levels. In 2012–2013, he was a member of the Chief Knowledge Officer's Public Health England Local Contribution Advisory Group. In addition to his membership of the UK Public Health Register, he is a member of the Local Area Research and Intelligence Association (LARIA) Council and the UK Health Statistics User Group (HSUG) Committee and also holds an honorary lectureship in health informatics at the Institute of Population Health, University of Manchester. Public Health, Manchester City Council, Manchester, UK

Isabelle Bray, Ph.D., M.Sc. is a senior lecturer in public health at the University of the West of England, UK. She has a background in medical statistics and epidemiology and has worked in several universities, central government and in an international health research institute. Current teaching interests include quantitative research methods and critical appraisal skills. Issy's research interests include cancer epidemiology and the relationships between mental health and physical activity. University of the West of England, Bristol, UK

Adam Briggs, M.A., B.M.B.Ch., M.Sc. is a Wellcome Trust Research Training fellow and honorary specialty registrar in public health at the University of Oxford, UK. He trained in medicine, specialising in public health, and is studying for a D.Phil. modelling the cost-effectiveness of public health policies. He enjoys teaching and his research interests include non-communicable disease prevention and examining the relationships between diet, health and sustainability. University of Oxford, Oxford, UK

Susan Cliffe, Ph.D., M.P.H. is a public health epidemiologist. She has more than 20 years of experience in academic and research work, which includes communicable disease surveillance at Public Health England, London School of Hygiene and Tropical Medicine and University of New South Wales. Her research interests are wide ranging, although she has a special focus on HIV/STI surveillance.

Jacqui Dorman, B.Sc., Pg.Dip., M.Sc. is a public health manager at Tameside Metropolitan Council, Greater Manchester, UK. She has nearly 10 years of experience in public health intelligence, which includes contributions to public health intelligence teaching, mentoring and training. Her interests are varied but her focus areas of work are related to reducing health inequalities and promoting the use of evidence and intelligence in all decision-making processes across the health and social care system. Tameside MBC, Oldham, UK

Julian Flowers, M.R.C.P., F.F.P.H., B.A. is a public health consultant and head of Public Health Data Science in Public Health England. He has a clinical background in general internal medicine and has spent the last 10 years working and developing public health intelligence in the NHS and in Public Health England. Public Health England, Cambridge, UK

Ivan Gee, Ph.D., M.Sc. is a senior lecturer in public health at the Centre for Public Health, Liverpool John Moores University. He has considerable experience in public health and in particular public health intelligence, having run an M.Sc. programme specifically focusing on public health intelligence. He contributes to teaching at master's and degree levels and has been involved in programme administration. He has a range of research interests relating to the impact of environmental factors on health and has worked in particular on the control of second-hand tobacco smoke. Liverpool John Moores University, Liverpool, UK

Ruth Gilbert, Ph.D. is a senior lecturer in public health at the University of Bedfordshire. She has more than 20 years of experience in academic and research work, including developing and undertaking communicable disease surveillance at Public Health England. Ruth has researched and published on a wide range of health protection-related issues, with a special focus on population-based infectious disease surveillance. University of Bedfordshire, Luton, UK

Alison Hill, B.Sc., F.F.P.H., F.R.C.P. (Lon.) is a public health consultant with Better Value Healthcare Ltd., leading the public health workstream and directing the Critical Appraisal Skills Programme. She is an honorary senior lecturer at Oxford University. Until July 2014 she was Public Health England's deputy chief knowledge officer. Previously she was managing director of Solutions for Public Health, an NHS business unit, providing highly specialised public health evidence and intelligence services to the NHS and local government. Better Value Healthcare Ltd., Oxford, UK

Katie Johnson, BSc, PGDip, MPhil, MFPH is a specialty registrar in public health working in the East of England. She has a background in local government and has worked in a variety of public health settings including local and regional health commissioning, health protection and public health intelligence. Norfolk and Norwich University Hospitals NHS Foundation Trust, Norwich, UK

Kristen Kurland, BA is Teaching Professor of Architecture, Information Systems, and Public Policy at Carnegie Mellon University's H. John Heinz III College and School of Architecture. Professor Kurland's research focuses on interdisciplinary collaborations in health, the built environment and spatial analysis using geographic information systems (GIS). Her teaching at CMU includes building information modelling (BIM), computer-aided design (CAD), 3D visualisation and GIS. At Heinz College, she also teaches infrastructure management to executive physicians in the master of medical management (MMM) programme and is a faculty advisor for Heinz College Health Care Management and Policy Systems Synthesis projects. She has a strong interest in technology-enhanced learning and has been teaching online courses since 1999. Professor Kurland is also the co-author of a series of best-selling GIS workbooks for Esri, Inc., the world's leading GIS software developer, including *GIS Tutorial 1 Basic Workbook*, *GIS Tutorial for Health* and *GIS Tutorial for Crime Analysis*. Carnegie Mellon University, Pittsburgh, PA, USA

Krishna Regmi, Ph.D., M.P.H., S.F.H.E.A., F.R.S.M., F.R.S.P.H. is a principal lecturer in public health and public health portfolio lead at the University of Bedfordshire. Over the past 24 years, he has been working in public health, undertaking a variety of course leadership, teaching and research responsibilities both internationally and in the UK. Over the last 3–4 years, he has been developing his interest in health intelligence and also runs a public health intelligence module at postgraduate level. His research interests are wide ranging, but he has a special focus on health system research, including primary healthcare, health sector reform, decentralisation, health inequalities and global health. University of Bedfordshire, Luton, UK

Peter Scarborough, D.Phil. is a university research lecturer at the University of Oxford. He has worked for more than 10 years in the field of public health related to diet, obesity and cardiovascular diseases and has published over 70 articles in peer-reviewed journals. His background is in mathematics and he was recently awarded a fellowship from the British Heart Foundation to develop novel mathematical models to predict cardiovascular disease burden in England. University of Oxford, Oxford, UK

Adrian Smith, M.B.B.S., M.Sc., D.Phil. is an associate professor at the University of Oxford. He qualified in medicine and specialised in infectious disease epidemiology. His research interests include epidemiology of HIV and STI in high-risk populations and imported malaria, and he has experience of generating primary data to model the impact of HIV prevention interventions in sub-Saharan Africa. University of Oxford, Oxford, UK

Colin Thunhurst, Ph.D., M.Sc., B.Sc. (Econ.) is an honorary principal research officer within the Faculty of Health and Life Sciences at Coventry University. He formally retired in 2008 after a 40-year career in the applied side of academia. Initially and for the first 20 years, he taught statistics and operational research, the subject of his first two degrees, with a specialist interest in health sector inequalities. He subsequently, and for the latter half of his career, made the substantive move into health sector management and public health, working particularly with developing health systems. During this period he has acted as health planning adviser to the Federal Government of Pakistan and has been project director for health sector projects in Pakistan and Nepal. He has worked as a short-term consultant to projects in numerous countries within Africa and Asia. Coventry University, Sandbeds, UK

Patrick Tobi, M.B.B.S., M.P.H., M.Sc., F.M.C.P.H. is a principal research fellow and head of research at the Institute for Health and Human Development, University of East London, UK. He is a public health physician with experience in public health practice, education and research in the UK and internationally. His interests lie at the interface between intervention programmes and the wider health and social systems in which they operate, with a particular focus on whole systems approaches and mixed methods programme evaluation. University of East London, Stratford, UK

Public Health Intelligence: An Overview

Krishna Regmi, Neil Bendel, and Ivan Gee

Public health without information is like pathology without a laboratory
Michael Goldacre

Abstract The notion that medical statistics could be used to assess and then identify potential risks or associated factors to be able to prevent avoidable human loss emerged sometime in the early seventeenth century (http://www.hsj.co.uk/Journals/2/Files/2010/5/24/APHO%20supplement.pdf). John Snow's work in studying the pattern of disease in order to trace the source of a cholera outbreak in London in 1854 established many of the concepts of modern epidemiology and demonstrated the link between data *analysis* and the necessary *action* to tackle the underlying causes of disease and ill health. More recently, the emergence of public health intelligence as a specific public health discipline is a response to the increasing recognition of the need to ensure that the development of appropriate strategies and policies to improve the health of the population and reduce health inequalities is underpinned by a rigorous and robust evidence base.

The manner in which public health intelligence has emerged as an accepted public health discipline means that it is not easy to identify a precise starting point or arrive at a commonly accepted definition. However, it is increasingly acknowledged that public health intelligence requires the application of a distinctive range and

K. Regmi (✉)
Faculty of Health and Social Sciences, University of Bedfordshire,
Putteridge Bury Campus, IHR-32, Luton LU2 8LE, UK
e-mail: Krishna.regmi@beds.ac.uk

N. Bendel
Public Health, Manchester City Council, PO Box 532, Level 4, Town Hall Extension,
Manchester M60 2LA, UK
e-mail: n.bendel@manchester.gov.uk

I. Gee
Center for Public Health, Liverpool John Moores University,
Henry Cotton Building, 15-21 Webster St, Liverpool L3 2ET, UK
e-mail: i.l.gee@ljmu.ac.uk

© Springer International Publishing Switzerland 2016
K. Regmi, I. Gee (eds.), *Public Health Intelligence*,
DOI 10.1007/978-3-319-28326-5_1

blend of analytic, critical and interpretive skills in order to generate meaningful information for decision-making. Many of the skills and techniques used to generate public health intelligence are shared with other domains of public health, such as epidemiology, and there is already a substantial body of literature and educational resources on these areas of practice. However, there is very little evidence and few resources available in the specific area of public health intelligence.

By the end of this chapter, you should be able to:

- Understand the concepts of public health and public health intelligence
- Explore the nature and roles of public health intelligence in measuring health and health outcomes of a defined population
- Examine some opportunities and challenging aspects of public health intelligence

Introduction

By way of introduction, it is useful to provide some historical background in order to track the gradual emergence and recognition of public health intelligence as a distinct and defined element of public health (see Box 1 below). Although this is largely drawn from a UK context, some of the key themes will be recognisable from a wider global perspective as well.

As Alison Hill and Julian Flowers note in "The Future Directions of Health Intelligence" chapter of this book, there is a long, strong and honourable tradition within public health of the use of evidence and information, going back to the nineteenth century. The notion that medical statistics could be used to assess and then identify potential risks or associated factors to be able to prevent avoidable human loss emerged sometime in the early seventeenth century (Donaldson 2010). John Snow's work in studying the pattern of disease in order to trace the source of a cholera outbreak in London in 1854 established many of the concepts of modern epidemiology. By using a spot map to illustrate how cases of cholera were centred on a public water pump, Snow was able to convince the parish authorities to take action to disable the well pump by removing its handle, thus eliminating the source of the outbreak. This demonstrated the link between data *analysis* and the necessary *action* to tackle the underlying causes of disease and ill health. This is described in more detail in "The Future Directions of Health Intelligence" chapter, which deals with some of the key issues in the presentation of data in public health intelligence.

In the Victorian era, the introduction of a national process for registering births, marriages and deaths in England and Wales in 1837, together with the emergence of the post of Medical Officer of Health in the mid nineteenth century (beginning with the appointment of William Henry Duncan as the Medical Officer of Health for Liverpool in 1847), provided a focal point for the systematic collection, reporting and presentation of data on communicable diseases and other causes of ill health in a local area. The Medical Officer of Health's Annual Report (the forerunner of today's Public Health Annual Report) remains an important source of historic public health data and analysis (see http://wellcomelibrary.org/moh/about-the-reports/about-the-medical-officer-of-health-reports/for more information).

Since the mid-1970s, and particularly since the introduction of the purchaser/provider split in 1991, both national and local NHS organisations have seen their roles and responsibilities increasingly defined in terms of their duty to address the health needs of local people through the effective commissioning of appropriate health services to meet these needs (PHE 2013; Bossert 1998). The NHS reorganisation of

---

Box 1. Key Milestones in the Emergence of Public Health Intelligence in England

1837—Introduction of a national process for registering births, marriages and deaths in England and Wales

1849—First Medical Officer of Health report (Sir John Simon's City of London Annual Report)

1854—John Snow's work on tracing the source of a cholera outbreak in London

1974—Establishment of Regional and District Health Authorities with a more clearly defined role in terms of assessing the needs of the population

1990—Establishment of Liverpool Public Health Observatory

1991—Publication of 'Purchasing Intelligence' report

2000—Launch of Public Health Observatories in England

2007—Publication of 'Informing Healthier Choices' strategy

2012—Health and Social Care Act. Establishment of Public Health England Knowledge and Intelligence Teams and transfer of public health responsibilities to local government

---

1974 led to the establishment of Regional and District Health Authorities with a more clearly defined role in terms of assessing the needs of the population and developing local services to meet these needs. The NHS and Community Care Act 1990, which led to the creation of an internal market in healthcare provision through the separation of the 'purchaser' and 'provider' functions of the NHS, helped to further this process by making health needs assessment (and the public health data and analysis underpinning it) one of the primary roles of the new purchasing authorities.

Looking beyond the UK, France established its first health observatories in 1974 to facilitate the decision-making process in health and social care by feeding appropriate intelligence through locating, identifying, assembling, analysing, criticising and synthesising of information to inform regional health policy (Hemmings and Wilkinson 2003).

The report 'Purchasing intelligence' published by the NHS Management Executive in 1991 described 'intelligence' as 'the full range of knowledge (text and numbers) needed for evidence-based decision-making' and was an early attempt to describe the concept of a local intelligence function and the sorts of information it might need to deal with. Many local areas responded to this report by developing new and innovative ways of delivering a public health intelligence function. The University of Liverpool established the first Public Health Observatory in 1990 with the aim of contributing to the development of appropriate health policies on the basis of relevant and accurate information (evidence-based intelligence) (Lewis et al. 2015; Wilkinson and Ferguson 2010). Across the North Western health region, a network of Public Health Research Centres (PHRCs) was established. Unlike the Public Health Observatory, each PHRC was embedded in an NHS organisation (rather than an academic institution) and sought to provide public health intelligence in the form of statistical data, research capability and public engagement skills relevant to public health in their local areas (Jones and Pickstone 2008).

The publication of a White Paper on public health ('Saving Lives: Our Healthier Nation') in 1998 was followed by the launch of a network of eight regional Public Health Observatories across England in 2000. This was symbolic in terms of bringing public health intelligence into the mainstream of national policy development.

The development and implementation of a comprehensive public health information and intelligence strategy was one of the commitments given in the White Paper 'Choosing Health'. Informing Healthier Choices (2007) was the first national strategy for improving the availability, timeliness and quality of health information and intelligence. This strategy emphasises four important areas of focus: workforce capacity and capability, improved data and information provision, stronger organisations, a health information and intelligence portal and underlying systems, with the notion that everyone with a responsibility for planning and commissioning services can do so on the basis of the best available knowledge.

The Health and Social Care Act 2012 gave upper tier and unitary local authorities in England a new statutory duty to improve the health of their populations, as well as a responsibility to provide public health advice on healthcare services to NHS commissioners and help ensure that plans are in place to protect the health of the population from outbreaks of infection or environmental hazards. A new national organisation (Public Health England) was tasked with actively supporting this work by engaging with local authorities to develop an effective knowledge and intelligence service and by leading on, or contributing to, relevant national policy and delivery.

In practice, this meant that many local authorities took over responsibility for existing public health intelligence teams and staff members that were previously employed by the NHS, in order to ensure that they had an effective source of health intelligence support to help them fulfil these significant new public health functions. The legal transfer of public health intelligence teams and their transition into local authority structures has largely been achieved successfully but a number of challenges remain, particularly in terms of the continued access to relevant NHS data and information.

Public Health Intelligence in Other UK Countries

The organisational arrangements for public health intelligence differ in each of the four parts of the UK. In addition to the arrangements in England described elsewhere in this chapter, the following national organisations are involved in providing public health intelligence in Scotland, Wales and Ireland:

- ScotPHO is a collaboration of key national organisations involved in public health intelligence and is led by the Information and Statistics Division (ISD) Scotland and NHS Health Scotland. See http://www.scotpho.org.uk/ for more information.
- The Public Health Wales Observatory is part of Public Health Wales. It aims to assist local and national partners by providing meaningful information to address public health issues, to improve health and health services and to reduce health inequalities. See http://www.publichealthwalesobservatory.wales.nhs.uk/ for more information.
- The Ireland and Northern Ireland's Population Health Observatory (INIsPHO) is housed within the Institute of Public Health in Ireland (IPH) and helps those working to improve health and reduce health inequalities by producing, disseminating and supporting the use of relevant health knowledge and strengthening the research and information infrastructure on the island of Ireland. It is unique in that it covers both the Republic of Ireland and Northern Ireland. See http://www. inispho.org/ for more information.

Unlike in England, the local public health function in **Scotland** is still part of the NHS, specifically, the 14 NHS Area Boards, and the local public health intelligence function also sits within the same set of organisations. However, as in England, the move towards greater integration of health and social care in Scotland through the creation of integrated health and social care partnerships means that this may change in the future (for more information, see http://www.gov.scot/Topics/Health/Policy/ Adult-Health-SocialCare-Integration). The Scottish Public Health Network provides links to a range of local public health reports by NHS Area Boards including Directors of Public Health (DPH) reports, lifestyle survey reports and other more specialised local reports (see www.scotphn.net/resources/local_health_intelligence_reports/).

In **Wales**, the current public health system is delivered through seven Health Boards, which are responsible for delivering all healthcare services within specified geographical areas. Public Health Wales provides each health board and the 22 local authorities in Wales with specialist public health support. The Welsh Government has issued a Public Health White Paper ('Listening to you—Your Health Matters') that sets out a series of proposals for legislation to help further improve and protect people's health and well-being in Wales. However, unlike in England, the Welsh proposals stop short of returning the public health system to local authorities.

In *Ireland*, the Health Services Executive (HSE) provides all of the country's public health services, in both hospitals and communities. Within the HSE, there are eight Departments of Public Health covering the Republic of Ireland, each providing Public Health expertise and services locally and nationally. Each Department is led by a Director of Public Health who is also the regional Medical Officer of Health. Knowledge management and health intelligence forms part of the organisational structure of the Health and Well-being Directorate within which Public Health is a partner.

What Is Public Health Intelligence?

The manner in which public health intelligence has emerged as an accepted public health discipline means that it is not easy to identify a precise starting point or arrive at a commonly accepted definition. The term 'intelligence' has been very much used within the context of UK health systems, although the meaning and its interpretations may vary across countries. The box below contains a range of different definitions of public health intelligence.

Looking further afield, the Australian National Public Health Partnership considers public health intelligence as the process of 'gathering and analysing information about the determinants of health, the causes of ill health and patterns and trends of health and ill health in the population' (National Public Health Partnerships 2006,

Definitions

The use of population information which has been analysed, interpreted and presented in clear and accessible form to inform proposed improvements to health services or to those factors which determine health, and which allow later examination to assess success (London Health Observatory 2006).

The systems and processes for assessing, measuring and describing health and well-being, including health needs and health outcomes of defined populations—drawing together of information from various sources in new ways to improve health and well-being Public Health Skills and Career Framework (PHORCAST 2013, also see Wright et al. 2008).

Public health information and intelligence covers a range of activities needed to support, inform, monitor and evaluate public health activities…it includes, but is not limited to, the collection of data, evidence from practice and outputs from research (information), analysis, evaluation and modelling (intelligence) and is obviously closely linked in some cases to direct action and/or to communication of outputs to influence the activity of others, such as commissioners of public health interventions (Public Health England 2011).

The process of understanding and analysis of public health information in support of population, healthcare planning and healthcare outcomes (Public Health England 2013).

p. 32). In a North American context, the phrase 'public health intelligence' has a more limited use than in the UK, with a tendency to interpret the meaning of intelligence primarily as the use of information for the purposes of early detection and response to infectious disease outbreak (Mordini and Green 2013; WHO 2005).

Dorman et al. (2009) state that public health intelligence 'uses statistical and epidemiological expertise to collate, analyse and interpret data to support public health and world class commissioning' (p. 5). This has aspects in common with the meaning of surveillance as used by WHO (2013), who define surveillance as the process of systematic, ongoing collection, collation and analysis of data and the timely dissemination of public health information for assessment and public health response as necessary (please refer to "Public Health Surveillance" chapter for the concept and key features of public health surveillance).

There are a number of common features running across all of these definitions:

- Public health intelligence requires a focus on both systems and processes
- Intelligence is generated through a *synthesis* of information drawn from a range of different sources and systems rather than an in-depth analysis of individual evidence or datasets
- Public health intelligence draws on a multiplicity of information sources and types, ranging from the determinants of health through to access to, and utilisation of, health and social care service and health outcomes
- The practice of public health intelligence spans the full intelligence 'cycle' or 'continuum'—from collection, generation, synthesis, appraisal, analysis, interpretation and communication
- Public health intelligence acts as a link between data analysis and action in terms of the provision of evidence to support improved decision-making, policy development and implementation

In the UK, the Public Health Skills and Knowledge Framework (PHORCAST 2013) has attempted to codify the skills and competencies required by the public health intelligence workforce and, in doing so, has helped public health intelligence to be recognised as a defined speciality within public health. The Framework (often called the 'PHRU-biks' cube) lists a range of core competencies, including the collection and collation of data on defined populations from a wide range of sources, analysis and interpretation of routine data using appropriate analytical techniques, presentation of the outcomes of data analysis in different ways to different audiences, support and provision of advice to others who are undertaking data collection, collation and analysis, and translation and communication of findings into appropriate recommendations for action (see Fig. 1).

The UK Faculty of Public Health (FPH) and Public Health Register (UKPHR) also view public health intelligence as a defined specialist area of public health practice in which professionals or practitioners are able to assess people's healthcare needs, analyse them, and offer appropriate and effective healthcare interventions to bring lasting change in people's health (Jenner et al. 2010; Wright et al. 2008).

Some authors claim that public health intelligence is a 'fourth' domain of public health—alongside healthcare, health protection and health improvement within public health, forging links between the fields of epidemiology, biostatistics and

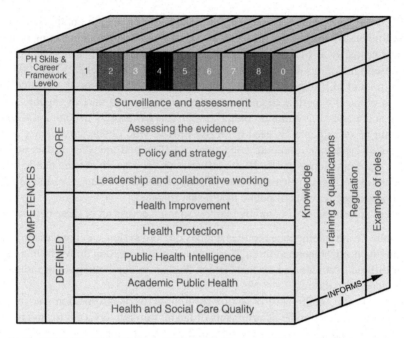

Fig. 1 The UK Public Health Skills and Knowledge Framework (*Source*: PHORCAST 2013)

public health—emphasising the increasing importance of making best use of intelligence to improve public health (Wilkinson 2007; PHE 2013).

However, in "The Future Directions of Health Intelligence" chapter of this book, Alison Hill and Julian Flowers argue that the way that these competencies have been articulated creates a distinct separation of the skills of finding and appraising evidence and handling data and information, and focuses insufficiently on knowledge translation. This requires an awareness of how knowledge is absorbed and acted on by users and hence an understanding of the behavioural sciences.

Discussion Task

Describe your understanding of public health intelligence; why/how does appropriate decision-making in public health practice require reliable health intelligence?

Comments: It is both the systems and process for assessing, measuring and describing the health and outcomes, and the intelligence is gained from synthesising the evidence. 'Intelligence' also relates to appropriate interpretation and inference of tailor-made information to make informed decisions. Public health intelligence is an intellectual process of moving through data to knowledge and intelligence continuum, in terms of exploring how intelligence is synthesised—gathered, analysed and translated into policy in practice.

Why Is Public Health Intelligence Important?

Over the past few decades, the discipline of public health or healthcare has greatly benefitted from the effective use of health information in assessing the health needs of the population, analysing and appraising potential health or health-related issues, and drawing some specific health actions in bringing lasting change in people's health status (Fu et al. 2009, p. 395). Pencheon et al. (2006) argue that 'if public health is the science and art of improving the health and populations, then measuring health status and assessing the health needs of populations are the universal starting points for most of its activities' (p. 78). As public health requirements are different and their needs are unique (Friede et al. 1994), our decisions will be determined by the degree of timely, reliable information available (AbouZahr and Boerma 2005). In other words, the information system is a core aspect of any public health activity. As Fu et al. (2009) point out, the purpose of public health information is the process of transferring data into information and then to intelligence at the stage where we can draw evidence-based decisions for action using evidence-based information.

Though the demand for information for health progress and impact of health services is increasingly global and 'data-intensive' (Evans and Stansfield 2003), certain health attributes—fertility and family planning and their impact on health and on the priority of areas such as maternal mortality—are difficult to measure, largely due to both the lack of reliable data and indicators, and the complexity (or diversity) of data and sources (Hill et al. 2001). Recently, health systems worldwide have been under pressure to generate, or develop, the health information—based on evidence and local intelligence—that is needed not only to make decisions and local actions, but also to be responsive to addressing changing healthcare needs of the population, which is a major obstacle to public health (Jenner et al. 2010; Boerma 2005a; Shaw 2005). As WHO (2005)) states, 'helping countries build and sustain health information is a challenge' (p. 565).

In the 1980s, information was heavily focused on clinical data and disease control and surveillance. However, in the 1990s, the focus shifted towards public health information, for example, the World Health Survey or Global Burden of Disease Study, which employed data and modelling to determine some major public health problems (WHO 2005; Boerma 2005a, b). In Scott's (2005) view, the purpose of health information systems is to identify health issues in order to inform health planning and design policy choices, as well as forecasting future health scenarios. Scott further argues that one way to address the problem is to promote health information systems that are appropriate to the infrastructure, technological capacity and budgets of health ministries. Appropriate decision-making in public health practice requires reliable health intelligence (useful information), otherwise '[…]decision-makers are unable to identify problems and needs and track progress, evaluate the impact of interventions and make evidence-based decisions on health policy, programme design and resource allocation' (Ashraf 2005, p. 565).

Public Health Intelligence in Practice

It has been widely acknowledged that knowledge and evidence-informed decision-making in health are critical. Health systems worldwide are increasingly recognising the importance of good quality local evidence and intelligence underpinning local action (Jenner et al. 2010) and there is a growing awareness of the need for more investment in health information systems (McGrail and Black 2005) in order to create the 'culture of evidence-based policy-making, help identify issues, inform the design and choice of policies, forecast the future, monitor policy implementation and evaluate policy impact' (Scott 2005 cited in Williams 2005 p. 564). Simply stated, appropriate decision-making in public health practice requires reliable and useable information and intelligence.

Public health intelligence is central to the process of making informed decisions based on appropriate and reliable evidence because it operates along the whole of the data-information-action intelligence (DIA) continuum—from data collection, through management and analysis, to interpretation, communication and action. This is illustrated in Fig. 2 (below).

In this model, 'data' is seen as a 'raw' object which does not provide reliable meaning per se but needs to be processed in order to turn it into meaningful 'information'. In turn, the production of 'intelligence' comes through the appropriate interpretation and inference of this information in order to 'add value' to the data and support informed decision-making (East Midlands Public Health Observatory 2012). This process requires statistical knowledge and skills to analyse the data using appropriate methods and techniques and provide safe, reliable advice about causes, risk and death and disease rates in a population using correct inferences. The quality of the intelligence provided depends on how the underlying data and information is gathered, analysed and interpreted.

In Scotland, NHS Dumfries and Galloway (2012) consider health intelligence as an 'inputs–outputs' configuration, meaning the output from the processes of analysing, interpreting and reporting information relating to health. Health Intelligence uses a variety of inputs including national datasets, local databases, national reports, research papers and other sources. The main role of heath intelligence is to support strategic and operational management in taking evidence-based decisions (Fig. 3).

By combining local information with other data from multiple sources and applying appropriate analysis, informatics, public health methodology, skills and interpretation, public health intelligence practitioners can help to assess and then examine the healthcare needs of service users and offer appropriate and quality services (Flowers and Ferguson 2010). Wilkinson (2007) notes that gathering and understanding evidence relevant to users' needs and interests, together with aligning the design and delivery of appropriate services, are key elements of service improvement. In the same vein, the Department of Health (2012a, b) argues that effective and robust use of local health intelligence is important, not only to discharge local public health functions but also to shape public health functions in a strategic way.

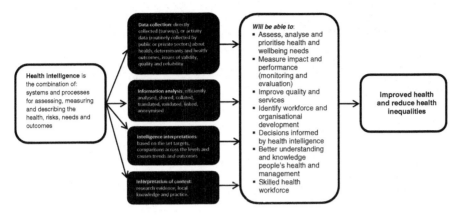

Fig. 2 Data-information-action continuum

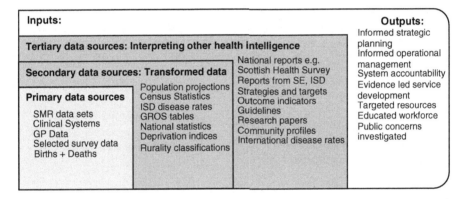

Fig. 3 Health intelligence 'input–output' figuration (*Source*: NHS Dumfries and Galloway 2012)

For this to happen, effective and sufficiently resourced public health intelligence teams need to be in place in order to be able to provide appropriate and relevant health evidence, as well as provision of specialist health intelligence skills and capability to deliver evidence informing performance in practice (Department of Health 2012a, b; Grey 2007).

Successive NHS reorganisations and other factors mean that the structures within which PHI operates are increasingly becoming more varied and the traditional model of PHI sitting with the public health department of a primary care trust (equivalent positions to the primary healthcare centre or district health office in several countries' health systems) is getting less common. Joint units within local government, including public health offices or local health authorities, are becoming more common, as are intelligence functions operating at sub-regional and regional healthcare levels. An example of this is the Kent Public Health Observatory (see below).

Case Study: Kent Public Health Observatory

The Kent Public Health Observatory provides public health intelligence and knowledge management support to Kent County Council, Clinical Commissioning Groups, district councils and other public sector organisations in Kent. The Observatory comprises two main teams: an Analytical Team responsible for the collation, analysis and dissemination of interpretable intelligence and, a Library and Knowledge Services team responsible for providing access to the latest public health research, books and journals to support public health and commissioning staff. The Library and Knowledge Services team also provide training in critical appraisal techniques literature review methods. The Observatory is funded directly via the Public Health Grant and is an integral part of the public health directorate. As such, the Observatory is a self-contained, dedicated resource for the public health directorate. The work programme is coordinated via the Head of Health Intelligence who is also a member of the senior management team, and the public health consultant team.

For more information on the work of the Observatory, please go to its website at http://www.kmpho.nhs.uk/.

Discussion Task

What are the key questions that might relate to accessing data in the early stages of health intelligence?

Comments:

- Who owns the data (data collector, national government or the community)?
- Who is responsible for data (ethical and legal issues, circumstances, storage and consent)?
- For what purposes will the data be used (programme planning and evaluation; what about beyond that, any subsequent use, or latitude for previously anticipated uses)?
- If the data will or may be used, what controls will be put in place to govern that use (do individuals or community require a say in what happens with the data; does a local representative need to be involved)?

Source: McGrail and Black (2005, p. 563)

Tools for Public Health Analysis

This book has 12 chapters altogether. Following an overview of public health intelligence (see chapter "Public Health Intelligence: An Overview"), the second chapter will focus more on the epidemiology and how it links to health intelligence (see chapter "Epidemiology and Public Health Intelligence"). Chapter "Types of Data and Measures of Disease" will describe the data, sources and appropriate measuring tools in assessing heath and healthcare needs. Chapter "Health Needs Assessment" will outline the concept of policy planning and evaluation, emphasising a whole systems approach to public health. The remaining chapters in this book will describe some of the key methodological, analytical and policy tools that are used by public health intelligence practitioners to inform and influence public health and wider health policy. The key features of these chapters have been given below.

In "Modeling in Public Health" chapter, Dr. Adam Briggs and colleagues from the University of Oxford outline the main uses and challenges of modelling in public health. They describe a range of situations in which public health modelling can be useful and discuss some of the key steps in building and interpreting a model, including highlighting how models can deal with assumptions and uncertainty. They also outline some of the main modelling methods, along with practical examples, and explain some of their limitations.

In "Public Health Surveillance" chapter, Ruth Gilbert from the University of Bedfordshire and Susan J. Cliffe describe how public health surveillance systems enable public health practitioners to assess and monitor changes in the population's health and make recommendations for action through the systematic, ongoing collection, analysis and dissemination of data. The chapter introduces some of the key concepts and objectives of public health surveillance and goes on to summarise the advantages and disadvantages of different surveillance systems. The authors conclude with a look at how advances in technology, social media and the internet are shaping the future of public health surveillance.

In "Geographic Information Systems in Health" chapter, Kristen Kurland from Carnegie Mellon University describes the use of geographic information systems (GIS) in public health. She provides an overview of the history and development of computerised GIS software and provides examples highlighting how the application of GIS tools and techniques can provide epidemiologists and others in the field of public health with tools to visualise, model and share health-related data. She goes on to discuss the future of GIS in terms of the integration of open source GIS, desktop, cloud-based tools and mobile devices and how social media and other means of collecting data offer new ways for public health practitioners to gain a better understanding of local communities.

Chapter "Synthesizing Public Health Evidence"—Ivan Gee from the LJMU and Krishna Regmi from the University of Bedfordshire discuss the methods and techniques of synthesising evidence. This chapter introduces the concept of research evidence, the process of synthesising research evidences and discusses how evidence informs decision-making in health and healthcare practice.

Chapter "Demography in Public Health Intelligence"—Patrick Tobi from the IIHD, University of East London, describes what a health needs assessment is and how it can be used to improve health and well-being. He goes on to discuss the range of approaches that currently influence thinking and practice underpinning health needs assessments.

In "The Future Directions of Health Intelligence" chapter, Dr. Julian Flowers and Katie Johnson from Public Health England discuss some of the key issues in the presentation of data in public health intelligence. They describe how data needs to be communicated in order to create insight or influence change and argue that visualisation and presentation of data in public health practice is a core—and increasingly important—skill. They go on to show how to select and create appropriate charts, discuss some of the new and developing tools that are available and give some examples of how data can influence policy and practice and demonstrate how visualisation can bring insight and clarity to this process.

In the UK, the establishment of a network of Public Health Observatories in the early 2000s has led to an expansion in the number of nationally produced public health analysis and visualisation tools, together with standard metadata and guidance on use (see, for example, Public Heath England's suite of national public health profiles on (http://fingertips.phe.org.uk/). There is also a greater range of commercially available products targeted towards public health intelligence uses.

In this context, much of the work of local public health intelligence practitioners is increasingly centred on 'knowledge translation', i.e. disseminating, adapting and interpreting the content of a range of tools in ways that make knowledge accessible and useable by the target user and in the context of locally determined strategic priorities and organisational structures. Typically, data from these tools are extracted, re-analysed and re-presented, along with other contextual information, and used as part of local population profiles, health needs assessments, equity audits, health/equality impact assessments, performance monitoring frameworks, predictive models and other local products. The use of local knowledge and intelligence in the context of the statutory Joint Strategic Needs Assessment (JSNA) is discussed in "Demography in Public Health Intelligence" chapter.

The skill of the local public health intelligence practitioner comes in understanding what data is available (and the pros and cons of that data), how it can be applied locally, and the best ways of getting the maximum impact from that data by ensuring that the right message is shared with the right people, in the right way and at the right time. While those working at regional or national levels aim to provide data and information which is current, accurate and openly accessible, people working at a local level invest significant effort in tailoring this information to generate health intelligence for local use: "We apply what is available at local level with our real understanding of the local population"; "We bring the right people together to use what we've got" (London Health Observatory 2006).

The Public Health Intelligence Workforce: Opportunities and Challenges

It has now been recognised that effective public health practice depends on access to the three planks of knowledge—intelligence, evidence and expertise—and that specialist public health intelligence skills and capacity are particularly needed now, when financial resources are limited. Does this represent a particular kind of shift for public health? If yes, what are the principles, resources and investments needed to ensure we have an adequate workforce?

A recent study of the public health knowledge and intelligence workforce by the Centre for Workforce Intelligence (CfWI) estimated that there are between 1070 and 1370 people working in a public health knowledge and intelligence role in England. However, the report also pointed out that there is no single, agreed definition covering what this workforce does. Given the increased focus on this element of the public health workforce, it will be important to have a clearer understanding of the size of the workforce, where staff are located and what their current and future professional needs are, in order to ensure effective delivery of public health knowledge and intelligence services (Centre for Workforce Intelligence 2015).

The CfWI report highlighted the increasing recognition of the role that this workforce plays in providing and developing a strong evidence base around public health and noted the extent to which the services offered by public health knowledge and intelligence teams are appreciated by local authority staff and others. Despite the growth of nationally produced tools and systems, Public Health England have acknowledged that 'Local intelligence support (e.g. in local authorities) should remain the first port of call for local intelligence enquiries' (Public Health England 2013). However, at the same time, the CfWI acknowledged a growing degree of uncertainty surrounding public health knowledge and intelligence—specifically within local authorities—as teams are reorganised and previously ring-fenced public health funding is potentially removed.

In "The Future Directions of Health Intelligence" chapter, Alison Hill and Julian Flowers discuss the future direction of health intelligence in the context of rapid developments in digital technology and the emergence of big data (and its associated new discipline of data science) and suggest how this might drive changes in public health intelligence. They also look at the global, national and local systems that are required for public health professionals to undertake their roles effectively and efficiently and what this means for the future in terms of the blend of skills that the new public health intelligence workforce require in order to take advantage of the changing nature of public health knowledge. In conclusion, they argue that there is a compelling and urgent need to rethink the training and development of this particular workforce to support them in taking up the extraordinary opportunities that are emerging within the field of public health knowledge.

The recent publication of a new PHE Workforce Strategy has highlighted the importance of developing the public health intelligence workforce as part of an integrated public health intelligence system in order to build knowledge and intelligence capacity at local, regional and national levels and support practitioners and decision-makers to make the best use of the available evidence in shaping public health policy and practice. However, as the CfWI has noted, there is currently no single national route for the professional accreditation and training of the public health intelligence workforce. The future for professional development may lie less in formal qualifications and more in training courses or schemes that develop professionals throughout their careers. The CfWI have recommended the development of a national professional network and an identifiable 'Head of Profession' for staff working in public health knowledge and intelligence functions in order to provide greater visibility and foster a stronger sense of community across this diverse workforce. Promoting career progression and workforce mobility between different organisations (e.g. Public Health England and local authorities) could help to reduce the possible risk of career stagnation and allow professionals to gain experience elsewhere where desired.

Conclusion

This chapter has highlighted that data, information and intelligence are at the heart of public health practice, and appropriate decision-making in public health practice requires reliable health intelligence (useful information). Lee (2003) pointed out that 'Health information is the glue that holds a health system together'. Health systems have now recognised the importance of basing local action on evidence and local intelligence from the perspectives of information related to provisions and services and population-based information.

> The '[p]ublic will benefit from this forethought if quality, useful datasets are developed and then made available for subsequent analysis that can provide guidance to improve health and healthcare'
>
> McGrail and Black (2005, p. 563)

References

AbouZahr, C., & Boerma, T. (2005). Health information systems: The foundations of public health. *Bulletin of the World Health Organization, 83*(8), 578–583.

Ashraf, H. (2005). Countries need better information to receive development aid. *Bulletin of the World Health Organization, 83*(8), 565–566.

Boerma, T. (2005a). Cost and results of information systems for health and poverty indicators in the United Republic of Tanzania. *Bulletin of the World Health Organization, 83*(8), 569–577.

Boerma, T. (2005b). Getting the numbers right. *Bulletin of the World Health Organization, 83*(8), 567–568.

Bossert, T. (1998). Analysing the decentralisation of health systems in developing countries: Decisions space, innovation and performance. *Social Science and Medicine, 47*(105), 1513–1527.

Centre for Workforce Intelligence. (2015). *The public health knowledge and intelligence workforce. A CfWI study*. London: Centre for Workforce Intelligence.

Department of Health. (1990a). *National Health Service and Community Care Act 1990*. London: HMSO. Retrieved September 26, 2015, from http://www.legislation.gov.uk/ukpga/1990/19/contents.

Department of Health. (1999b). *Saving lives: Our healthier nation*. London: HMSO. Retrieved September 14, 2015, from http://webarchive.nationalarchives.gov.uk/+/www.dh.gov.uk/en/Publicationsandstatistics/Publications/PublicationsPolicyAndGuidance/DH_4118614.

Department of Health. (2007). *Informing healthier choices: Information and intelligence for healthy populations*. (Gateway ref 8002) London: Department of Health. Retrieved September 14, 2015, from http://webarchive.nationalarchives.gov.uk/20130107105354/http://www.dh.gov.uk/prod_consum_dh/groups/dh_digitalassets/documents/digitalasset/dh_075485.pdf.

Department of Health. (2012a). *Factsheet: Local public health intelligence*. London: Department of Health.

Department of Health. (2012b). *Health and Social Care Act*. London: Department of Health.

Donaldson, L. (2010). Richer than ever in data. *Health Service Journal Supplement—27 May 2010*. Retrieved September 2, 2015, from http://www.hsj.co.uk/Journals/2/Files/2010/5/24/APHO%20supplement.pdf.

Dorman, J., McCormack, A., & Carroll, P. (2009). *Public Health Intelligence e-handbook*. Retrieved September 11, 2015, from http://s3.amazonaws.com/zanran_storage/www.gmphnetwork.org.uk/ContentPages/2481152558.pdf.

East Midlands Public Health Observatory. (2012). *Training and development of and Lettuce public health intelligence online 2012*. Retrieved September 2, 2015, from www.empho.org.uk/THEMES/phi/training.aspx

Evans, T., & Stansfield, S. (2003). Health information in the new millennium: A gathering storm? *Bulletin of the World Health Organization, 81*, 856.

Flowers, J., & Ferguson, B. (2010). The future of public health intelligence: Challenges and opportunities. *Public Health, 124*, 274–277.

Friede, A., Rosen, D. H., & Reid, J. A. (1994). CDC wonder: A cooperative processing architecture for public health. *Journal of the American Medical Informatics Association, 1*, 303–312.

Fu, P., Luck, J., & Protti, D. (2009). Information systems in support of public health in high-income countries. In R. Detels, R. Beaglehole, M. Lansang, & M. Gulliford (Eds.), *Oxford textbook of public health* (pp. 395–426). Oxford, England: Oxford University Press.

Grey, S. (2007). Academic public health. In S. Griffith & D. Hunter (Eds.), *New perspectives in public health*. Oxford, England: Radcliffe.

Hemmings, J., & Wilkinson, J. (2003). What is a public health observatory? *Journal of Epidemiology and Community Health, 57*, 324–326.

Hill, K., AbouZahr, C., & Wardlow, T. (2001). Estimates of maternal mortality for 1995. *Bulletin of the World Health Organization, 79*, 182–193.

Jenner, D., Hill, A., Greenacre, J., & Enock, K. (2010). Developing the public health intelligence workforce in the UK. *Public Health, 124*, 248–252.

Jones, E., & Pickstone, J. (2008). *The quest for public health in Manchester. The industrial city, the NHS and the recent history*. Manchester: Manchester NHS Primary Care Trust.

Lee, J. W. (2003). *Address to WHO staff*. Geneva: WHO. Retrieved September 3, 2015, from http://www.who.int/dg/lee/speeches/2003/21_07/en/

Lewis, C., Ubido, J., Roper, L., & Scott-Samuel, A. (2015). *An overview of the history and work of Liverpool Public Health Observatory, and its impact on policy and services. LPHO Report Series, number 103*. Liverpool: Liverpool Public Health Observatory. Retrieved September 11, 2015, from https://www.liv.ac.uk/media/livacuk/instituteofpsychology/publichealthobservatory/June,2015,LPHO,revised,overview.pdf.

London Health Observatory. (2006). *Mapping health intelligence and its dissemination in London: Summary findings*. Retrieved January 9, 2016, from http://www.lho.org.uk/viewResource.aspx?id=10898.

McGrail, K. M., & Black, C. (2005). Access to data in health information systems. *Bulletin of the World Health Organization, 83*(4), 563 [Editorials].

Mordini, E., & Green, M. (2013). *Internet-based intelligence in public health emergencies: Early detection and response in disease outbreak crisis*. Lansdale, PA: Ios Press.

National Public Health Partnerships. (2006). *Public health classifications project phase 1: Final report*. Melbourne, VIC, Australia: NPHP.

NHS Dumfries & Galloway. (2012). *Health intelligence unit operation plan*. Retrieved September 2, 2015, from http://www.nhsdg.scot.nhs.uk/dumfries/files/health_intelligence_operational_plan.pdf.

NHS Management Executive. (1991). *Purchasing intelligence*. London: NHS Management Executive.

Pencheon, D., Guest, C., Melzer, D., & Gray, M. (2006). *Oxford handbook of public health practice*. Oxford, England: Oxford University Press.

PHORCAST. (2013). *UK public health skills and knowledge framework*. London: PHORCAST.

Public Health England. (2011). *Public health England's operational model*. London: Department of Health.

Public Health England. (2013). *Knowledge and intelligence: Public Health England's local contribution to the work of local government and the NHS*. London: PHE.

Scott, C. (2005). *Measuring up to the measurement problem the role of statistics in evidence-based policy-making*. Retrieved July 4, 2015, from http://www.paris21.org/sites/default/files/1509.pdf.

Shaw, V. (2005). health information system reform in South Africa: Developing an essential data set. *Bulletin of the World Health Organization, 83*(8), 632–636.

Simon, J. (1848-1849). *Report on the sanitary condition of the City of London for the year 1848-9*. Retrieved September 9, 2015, from http://wellcomelibrary.org/player/b1824404x#?asi=0&ai=0.

Wilkinson, J. (2007). Public health intelligence and public health observatories. In S. Griffiths & D. Hunter (Eds.), *New perspectives in public health*. Oxford, England: Radcliffe.

Wilkinson, J., & Ferguson, B. (2010). The first initial public health observatories in England and the next? *Public Health, 124*, 245–247 [Editorial].

Williams, T. (2005). Building health information systems in the context of national strategies for the development of statistics. *Bulletin of the World Health Organization, 83*(8), 564 [Editorial].

World Health Organisation. (2005). Countries need better information to receive development aid. *Bulletin of the World Health Organization, 83*(8), 565–566.

World Health Organisation. (2013). *Public health surveillance*. Geneva, Switzerland: WHO.

Wright, J., Rao, M., & Walker, K. (2008). The UK public health skills and career framework— Could it be help to make public help the business of every workforce? *Public Health, 122*, 541–544.

Recommended Reading

Centre for Workforce Intelligence. (2015b). *The public health knowledge and intelligence workforce. A CfWI study*. London: Centre for Workforce Intelligence.

Dorman, J., McCormack, A., & Carroll, P. (2009). *Public Health Intelligence e-handbook: A guide for the public health analyst and wider workforce*. Manchester: Greater Manchester Public Health Intelligence Network. Retrieved September 11, 2015, from http://s3.amazonaws.com/zanran_storage/www.gmphnetwork.org.uk/ContentPages/2481152558.pdf.

World Health Organisation. (2014). *Providing health intelligence to meet local needs: A practical guide to serving local and urban communities through public health observatories*. Geneva, Switzerland: WHO.

Epidemiology and Public Health Intelligence

Isabelle Bray and Krishna Regmi

> *Epidemiology* is the study of the distribution and determinants of health-related states or events in specified populations and the application of this study to the control of health problems.
>
> *From Last 2001—Dictionary of Epidemiology*

Abstract This chapter provides an introduction to epidemiology. It covers the key epidemiological concepts such as bias and confounding, as well as providing an overview of the nature, history and types of epidemiology. The main epidemiological study designs are described, including case series, ecological, cross-sectional, case–control, cohort, randomised controlled trial and systematic review. The advantages and disadvantages of each are summarised, and some of the ethical issues in doing research are considered. The 'hierarchy of evidence' framework is contrasted with an approach which recognises the most appropriate study design to answer different questions about population health. This chapter will examine the role of epidemiology in public health intelligence and develop students' or learners' knowledge and skills to carry out thorough, rigorous and meaningful research and investigation relevant to public health.

After reading this chapter you should be able to:

- Define epidemiology and differentiate between descriptive epidemiology and analytical epidemiology
- Describe the basic study designs, principles and methods used in epidemiology
- Explore key issues related to the design and conduct of studies
- Recognise the role of epidemiology in public health intelligence

I. Bray (✉)
Department of Health and Social Sciences, Faculty of Health and Applied Sciences,
University of the West of England, Frenchay Campus, Coldharbour Lane,
Bristol BS16 1QY, UK
e-mail: issy.bray@uwe.ac.uk

K. Regmi
Faculty of Health and Social Sciences, University of Bedfordshire,
Putteridge Bury Campus, IHR-32, Luton LU2 8LE, UK

© Springer International Publishing Switzerland 2016
K. Regmi, I. Gee (eds.), *Public Health Intelligence*,
DOI 10.1007/978-3-319-28326-5_2

19

What Is Epidemiology?

Descriptive epidemiology is concerned with both the frequency and distribution of a health outcome (or health-related exposure). In other words, how common is it, and who does it affect? The first question can be answered using measures such as incidence and prevalence (see "Types of Data and Measures of Disease" chapter). The second can be framed in terms of TIME, PLACE and PERSON (see Fig. 1). For example, we may describe the distribution of health outcomes by age, population, geography or over time.

Descriptive epidemiological outputs are often presented graphically. Disease atlases and graphs showing trends over time are commonly used techniques to highlight disparities in health status between countries or areas within countries and to illustrate changes in health outcomes over time. These techniques are particularly important for highlighting inequalities according to not only geography, but also by age, gender, levels of deprivation, ethnicity and occupation. Many routine health reports present outcomes by quintiles of deprivation, and in New Zealand the Ministry of Health routinely reports on differences in health outcomes between the indigenous Maori population compared with the rest of the population (https://www.health.govt.nz/). It is quite common to see reported in the news maps showing outcomes such as life expectancy or quality of life for different regions or cities of the UK. Another important use of descriptive epidemiology is to monitor the incidence of new or rare diseases (examples include the global epidemics of bird flu and *ebola*). Maps (showing the number of cases recorded by region) and epidemic curves (plotting new cases against time) are tools often used in surveillance. See the "Public Health Surveillance" chapter for more information about health surveillance.

Analytical epidemiology, sometimes also known as aetiological epidemiology, considers the role of individual risk factors in the development of disease. In other words, investigating which factors are responsible for increasing or decreasing the risk of an outcome, and quantifying their effect. The key issue is to determine whether an exposure just happens to be associated with the outcome of interest, or whether it is causing the outcome (i.e. the association is causal). So while descrip-

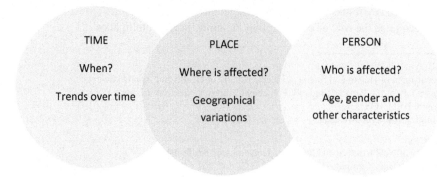

Fig. 1 Describing the distribution of disease

tive epidemiology may highlight a possible risk factor for a particular health outcome (e.g. suicide rates are increasing at the same rate as selective serotonin reuptake inhibitor (SSRI) prescribing, or immigrants are more likely to give birth to preterm babies than other women in the population), analytical epidemiology is used to determine what is actually causing the health outcome. Perhaps, for example, the rise in SSRI prescriptions has coincided with a decrease in funding for community mental heath services, and this is more directly related to suicide deaths. Or perhaps immigrant mothers are more likely to fall into age brackets associated with an increased risk of preterm birth, and this is the causal factor rather than immigrant status per se. These issues can be untangled through analytical epidemiology, with adequate control for confounding factors.

> **Confounding factors** are those which are related to both the exposure and outcome of interest, and which distort the association being studied.

Rigorous analytical epidemiology can be summarised by the 5 Ws (see Fig. 2). The TIME, PLACE and PERSON of descriptive epidemiology translate into WHEN, WHERE and WHO, respectively. To these can be added WHAT and WHY, i.e. what is the health outcome of interest and why does it occur (e.g. what are the causes?)? The 5 Ws can be applied when considering any health condition in a population, whether it be norovirus aboard a cruise ship or asthma amongst school children.

> **Discussion Task**
> What are the key terms in the definition of epidemiology?

The Changing Nature of Epidemiology

In his treatise '*On Airs, Waters, and Places*', Hippocrates (460BC–377BC) recognised the importance of the environment in the causation of disease. Epidemiology as a discipline developed in the area of infectious disease control, through the statistical analysis of routine data to quantify the risk associated with unsanitary environments (see, for example, the work of pioneer epidemiologists John Snow (1855) and William Farr (Ratcliffe 1974)). The epidemiology of communicable disease, and its application to Public Health, is sometimes also known as 'Health Protection' (something of a misnomer given that all epidemiology is about protecting health through identifying and limiting exposure to risk factors). Environmental epidemiology also includes, for example, studying the effect of pollution on the prevalence of asthma amongst children, and the health effects of environmental tobacco smoking. But

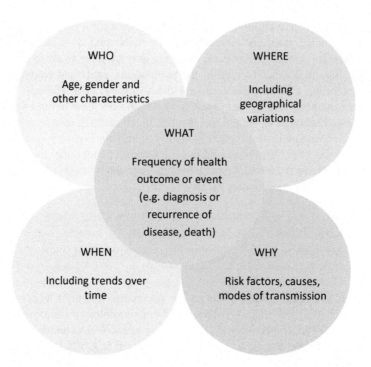

Fig. 2 The 5 Ws of analytical epidemiology

elucidating the causes of non-communicable diseases such as asthma, coronary heart disease and cancer is, by definition, harder than studying infectious diseases because there are a range of complex factors which may be causally related to the non-communicable disease in question, and possibly interactions between these factors.

One way to conceptualise epidemiology is as follows. Imagine you walk into a room; there is one switch on the wall, and you discover that this switch turns the light on and off. In the next room, there are several switches, but you find that only one of them controls the light. In a third room, there are also several switches, but none of them operates the light. You discover though trial and error that only a certain combination of these switches will turn the light on. In the final room, there are many switches on the wall and you find that *certain combinations* of switches will turn on the light, *some of the time*. In this scenario, the switches are the various exposures we are interested in (which may be environmental, genetic or behavioural), and the light is the disease outcome of interest. And so it is that we seek to understand the component causes of disease—why some people develop cancer and others not, why some children develop obesity and others not and why some people born into adversity have good health outcomes while others do not.

In the developed world, non-communicable disease has overtaken communicable disease as a priority. This is known as the *epidemiological transition*. The transition is partly due to the success of prevention measures put in place against infectious disease, and epidemiology still has an important role to play in providing evidence to support these measures (e.g. Madsen et al. 2002). Many developing countries going through the epidemiological transition are suffering a double burden, with high rates of infectious disease (e.g. malaria, HIV) and infant mortality due to preventable infectious disease, and at the same time a developing economy leading to more 'Westernised' lifestyles which brings with it increasing prevalence of non-communicable diseases such as cardiovascular disease and cancer. We note that despite our attempts to class diseases as being either communicable or non-communicable, we are increasingly discovering that conditions traditionally thought of as non-communicable can be associated, in part, with certain infections. Examples include *H. pylori* infection and coronary heart disease, hepatitis and liver cancer, and human papilloma virus and cervical cancer.

Just as a certain proportion of cancer cases can be attributed to infectious agents, other cases are due to genetic causes. *Genetic epidemiology* examines the role of genes in the development of diseases (e.g. breast cancer), and what are known as *gene–environment interactions*. This is when a certain combination of genetic predisposition and environmental exposure (e.g. to stress or a toxin) increase the risk of a certain health outcome occurring in an individual. *Epigenetic epidemiology* is concerned with environmental effects on the expression of genes rather than the DNA itself. We can think of genes being switched on or off by exposures experienced at critical periods (e.g. in utero or in the pre-pubertal slow growth period). For more about epigenetics, see '*The Epigenetics Revolution*' (Nessa Carey 2012). Epigenetic epidemiology takes us beyond the nature–nuture (gene–environment) dialogue and into a new dimension in which the environment can alter the expression of genes in such a way that the effects of environmental exposures on genes are passed down from one generation to the next. The discovery that our environment can have this effect on our genetic make-up, previously thought to be down to a roll of the dice at conception and then fixed, to be passed onto the next generation, emphasises the importance of environmental influences on health and well-being, and brings us full circle back to Hippocrates.

Epidemiological Study Designs

Epidemiological study designs can be categorised as being either observational (we study what is already happening, without intervening) or experimental (when we conduct a trial to assess the effects of an intervention on the health outcome of interest). In observational study designs, we want to quantify the effect of an exposure (e.g. environmental, genetic or behavioural) on the outcome, whereas in experimental study designs we are testing a potential intervention or treatment—in this case, the intervention is the exposure of interest. Since different terms are sometimes used interchangeably, or by different disciplines to mean the same thing, Fig. 3 lists various terms that may be used when talking about exposures and health outcomes in epidemiological research.

Within the broad categories of observational and experimental, there are several different study designs. These are sometimes thought of in terms of a 'hierarchy of evidence'. Although this approach has somewhat lost favour as over-simplifying the situation, it is still a useful framework for describing epidemiological study designs. Figure 4 lists the main study designs which will be considered here, ranging from case series to systematic review. These can be classified according to whether they are observational or experimental study designs, and also according

Context	Exposure	Health Outcome
Observational designs	Exposure	(Health) Outcome
	Risk factor	
Experimental designs	Treatment	Disease
	Intervention	Condition
Statistical modelling	Independent variable	Dependent Variable
	Explanatory factor	
	x	y

Fig. 3 Alternative terms used for exposures and health outcomes

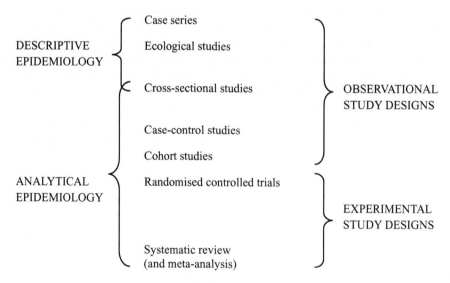

Fig. 4 The hierarchy of evidence showing the main epidemiological study designs, ordered from the least reliable (case series) up to the most reliable (systematic review)

to whether they are used for descriptive or analytical epidemiology. Of course, there are different versions of this framework, and other study designs could be included.

Case Series

A case series is a report on a number of cases exhibiting a similar set of symptoms, possibly describing a new syndrome. It is compiled from individual case reports and may lead to formulation of a new hypothesis relating to risk factors and disease. However, since it does not involve a control group and provides no evidence of a causal relationship, it can only suggest possibilities for further research. Our first example of a case series is a report called 'Thalidomide and congenital abnormalities' (McBride 1961). The author had noticed a number of babies with abnormal limbs being born to mothers who had taken thalidomide for morning sickness, and suspected a connection. His paper was published in The Lancet, and soon other doctors around the world were responding that they had noticed similar cases amongst their patients. This enabled a rapid response to prevent the drug being given to more pregnant women. The second example is more infamous—that is the case series that suggested a link between the MMR vaccination and autism (Wakefield et al. 1998). The case series was based on only 12 children. In fact, the paper itself (now retracted by the Lancet) was relatively cautious and the title does not even mention the vaccination. The conclusion contained the following statements—'*In most cases, onset of symptoms was after measles, mumps and rubella immunisation*' and '*Further investigations are needed to examine this syndrome and its possible relation to this vaccine.*' The second of these statements is appropriate to the limitations of a case series, but the misinterpretation of the first and its effect on MMR immunisation rates in many countries is well-documented elsewhere (Tannous et al. 2014). What is probably less well known is that the hypothesis was subsequently investigated by large cohort studies which showed no evidence of a link between the MMR vaccine and autism (e.g. Madsen et al. 2002).

Cross-Sectional Study

The defining feature of a cross-sectional study is that it is carried out at one point in time. A sample is drawn from the population of interest, and data collection is often through self-completed survey but may be through interviewer-administered questionnaire. This study design is ideal for descriptive epidemiology, in particular for estimating the prevalence of a given health condition (the proportion of the population who have the condition), or indeed the prevalence of an important exposure (such as smoking), but cannot measure incidence (the number of new cases in a given time period such as a year). Its appropriateness for analytical epidemiology is very limited by the fact that exposures are measured at the same time as disease outcomes, which creates a 'chicken and egg' problem. Imagine a survey that collects information on levels of physical activity and mental health, amongst other things. If there is a positive association between these variables, are we to conclude that physical activity improves mental health? Or might it be that people with better mental health are more likely to be motivated to take exercise? Other common problems with cross-sectional studies are low response rates which can lead to a non-representative sample (affecting the generalisability of the findings), and the measurement of exposure and outcome through self-report which can lead to reporting bias. For example, it is well known that people tend to under-report their tobacco and alcohol use, and a recent study found that men tended to over-report levels of physical activity (Dyrstad et al. 2013).

Bias is a systematic error in the measurement of the exposure or outcome variables.

Ecological Study

An ecological study is a cross-sectional study with the unit of analysis being a geographical area (e.g. a country, region or ward) rather than the individual (as is usual in epidemiology). Associations between potential exposures and the outcome of interest are often shown on a scatter graph, with each point representing a country (or other unit of analysis). Ecological studies suffer from the same drawbacks as other cross-sectional surveys when used for analytical purposes (confounding, exposure measured at the same time as outcome, bias in reporting of exposures and outcomes), but there is also the additional problem of the ecological fallacy. This means that associations that hold at a population level do not hold at an individual level. Take, for example, a study of average income and rates of coronary heart disease in capital cities of the world. This would show that those cities with the highest average income also had the highest rates of coronary heart disease, from which you might deduce that increased wealth is associated with increased risk of coronary heart disease. But, for Westernised societies at least, the opposite is true. If you look at individuals within wealthy cities such as London and Washington, it is the poorer people who have the highest rates of coronary heart disease. This is the ecological fallacy. However, ecological studies are often quick and easy to carry out since they can be conducted using routinely collected and often freely available data, and they are very useful for generating hypotheses to be tested in further more rigorous studies. For example, using dietary information from international studies and cancer incidence rates available by country from the WHO, you could carry out an ecological analysis to generate hypotheses about dietary risk factors for cancer. Another example of an ecological analysis is the *The Spirit Level* (Wilkinson and Pickett 2010), which examines income inequalities in a wide range of countries across the globe, and examines the association between this exposure and many health and social outcomes.

Case–Control Study

A case–control study (see Fig. 5) compares a group of people with a condition (the cases) with a similar group of people who do not have the condition (the controls). Cases and controls are drawn from the same population. The aim is to identify the risk factors which caused the condition, by comparing the exposure status of cases and controls. In order to ensure that any differences are not due to confounding factors such as age and gender, controls are usually selected to be similar to cases in these respects. This is called 'matching'. Other variables such as socio-economic status may also be matched upon. A case–control approach is particularly useful when we need to conduct a study quickly to ascertain the cause of a disease or health outcome. It could have been used, for example, following the thalidomide case series described above, to get more concrete evidence of the link, and it is also widely used to investigate infectious disease outbreaks.

A key aspect of this study design is that we are collecting exposure data retrospectively. This has disadvantages in terms of the reliability of that data, particularly if exposures are self-reported. The scale of the problem depends on what we are asking people to recall and the time that has elapsed since exposure. So if, for example, we were asking participants to report how many children they had given birth to, or whether they had been swimming in the previous week, we would hope that their memory of these exposures would be accurate. But if we ask participants to report how many tetanus vaccinations they had received before the age of 16, or how many coffees they had drunk in the last week, then this would be less reliably reported. Added to this general problem of less-than-perfect memories is recall bias which is usually the most serious drawback of using a case–control approach. It occurs because the exposures reported by cases and controls are biased by the very

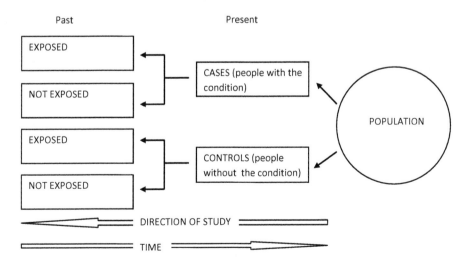

Fig. 5 Case–control study design

fact of being a case or control. People who have the health condition of interest may over-report potential risk factors, because they are trying to understand why they developed the condition, and looking to past exposures for reasons. Conversely, people who do not have the condition are likely to under-report exposures as they have no particular incentive to recall them, and their memory has faded with time. Of course, these are generalisations and the effect of recall bias will very much depend on the context and how the questions are asked, but recall bias is a very real phenomenon.

An example of this is a comparison between data on medical x-ray exposure obtained a) from medical records and b) from mailed questionnaires (Hallquist and Jansson 2005). In this case-control study of thyroid cancer, the authors concluded that both cases and controls underreported x-ray investigations, but that underreporting was of greater magnitude amongst the controls. The degree of underreporting was also found to differ according to age and gender. The authors concluded that recall bias was an important risk, if relying on self-report of x-ray exposure alone. Of course, if we are collecting data on exposures based on other data sources, such as medical records or other routinely available data, then recall bias is not a problem, but the suitability of the data for research purposes should be considered.

Cohort Study

A cohort study takes a group of people from the population of interest, measures exposures at the outset, and follows them up for a given period of time so that incidence of health outcomes can be ascertained (see Fig. 6). Many different exposures

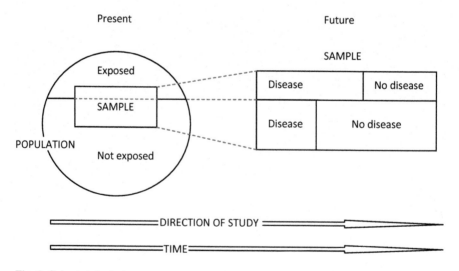

Fig. 6 Cohort study design

and outcomes can be considered. Exposure and outcome measurement may be through self-reported questionnaire, measured by observers (e.g. a research nurse at a clinic or during a home visit) or collected from existing data sources (e.g. educational or health records) through data linkage. Measurement of both exposures and outcomes may continue throughout follow-up.

Cohort studies can take many shapes and sizes. Some population-based studies follow up tens of thousands of participants for their entire lives. Data on a large number of exposures and outcomes may be recorded. Others follow more specific populations for shorter periods of time, and may be designed to answer a more focused research question. For example, a small cohort of patients with a rare condition might be followed up for 5–10 years to collect data on prognosis. If a cohort study is designed to investigate a particular exposure, the sample may be selected on the basis of exposure status, to ensure that sufficient numbers of participants who have experienced the exposure are included. This is particularly useful if the exposure is rare, e.g. exposure to asbestos.

An example of a large population-based cohort study is the Avon Longitudinal Study of Parents and Children (ALSPAC). Information was collected from approximately 14,000 women throughout their pregnancy. Data was also collected from the children from birth and is ongoing. ALSPAC is now a multi-generational study of immense value for answering all kinds of research questions. However, ALSPAC serves to illustrate a major drawback of cohort studies with reasonably long follow-up periods, which is drop-out over time. This occurs because participants move, die, become uncontactable, or simply do not wish to continue in the study. As well as reducing the sample size, this increases bias in the sample, because those who drop out are different to those who remain in the study. Twenty-five years after the study started, response rates to ALSPAC questionnaires are now approximately 50 %. Those who were still contributing data at age 16–18 were more likely to be female than those who had dropped out, more likely to be of white ethnicity and less likely to have been eligible for free school meals (Boyd et al. 2013).

Another major problem with cohort studies is that of confounding. Imagine a cohort study designed to test a possible association between alcohol consumption (exposure) and risk of lung cancer (outcome). A simple approach would be to take a sample from the population and collect data on alcohol consumption at the outset. The follow-up period would have to be long enough for sufficient numbers of cases of lung cancer to be diagnosed. Then, based on a naïve analysis which ignores confounding factors, you may conclude that there is a positive association between alcohol consumption and lung cancer. However, this apparent association is actually due to smoking status (which is associated with both alcohol consumption and risk of lung cancer). If this confounding factor is also measured and taken into account in the analysis, then the association between alcohol consumption and lung cancer can be explained. This simple example illustrates the point, but the reality is that there are many confounding factors leading to spurious associations between exposures and outcomes in observational epidemiological studies. Some are obvious and easy to understand (e.g. age, gender), others less so (e.g. educational status). Data must therefore be collected on all potential confounders so that they can be taken into account during analysis. There are often many confounding factors that we have not even thought of, so cannot measure. And there are those that we are aware of but are difficult to define and measure (e.g. socio-economic status, adverse childhood circumstances). In this situation, we attempt to capture the confounding factor (through use of a deprivation index, for example) but since this is imperfect there will be 'residual confounding' that we have not managed to control for.

Discussion Task
What are the advantages and disadvantages of observational study designs?

Randomised Controlled Trials

The randomised controlled trial (RCT) is thought of as the 'gold standard' of research designs. It is the most reliable way to test the effectiveness of a treatment or intervention. Interventions can be classed as primary prevention (to reduce the risk of exposure) or secondary prevention (therapeutic interventions to alleviate symptoms, prevent recurrence or decrease risk of mortality). An example of primary prevention would be a smoking cessation intervention. An example of secondary prevention would be chemotherapy for breast cancer.

A trial is any experiment to test an intervention. So you give a group of patients a new treatment, and they get better. Can you claim that the treatment is a success? Maybe they would have got better anyway (the body often heals itself with time). So we need a control group, and a trial which compares patients on the new treatment with another group of patients receiving either standard treatment (if there is one) or no treatment. Now, if the patients on the treatment get better more rapidly than those in the other treatment group, then the new treatment appears to be a success. But someone might argue that this was because the patients in the new treatment group were somehow different, and more likely to do well. Perhaps their disease was less severe, or they were younger, or they had better access to healthcare? This is the reason for randomising participants to the two groups. If they are allocated to the two groups on a completely random basis, then factors that might influence the success of the intervention (such as age, gender, disease severity) are evenly distributed between the two groups by the play of chance. Now, any difference in outcome between the two groups is not down to confounding factors, so must be due to the actual treatment. The key advantage of RCTs over observational study designs is that by randomising participants we are comparing two groups who should be similar in terms of all confounding factors, even those we are unaware of. The process of conducting an RCT is described in Fig. 7.

But could the observed treatment effect be, at least in part, due to the placebo effect? The patients receiving the new intervention know they are getting the latest treatment. They expect to feel better, and they do feel better (the mind plays an important role in these matters). So, if possible, we need to conduct a trial in which

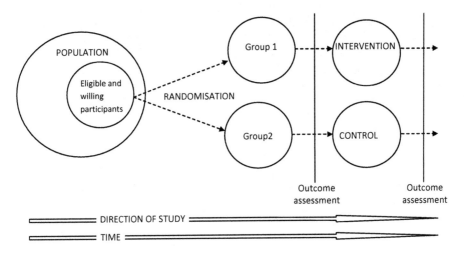

Fig. 7 Randomised controlled trial design

the participants do not know which treatment group they are in. This is known as 'blinding'. The participants in the study are 'blinded' to their treatment group. Then any self-reported outcomes, such as pain or quality of life, are not biased by knowledge of treatment group. Outcomes assessed by an observer (e.g. function scored by a physiotherapist) are also subjective and prone to bias, so observers should also be blinded. It is not always possible to blind participants and observers, depending on the intervention in question, but it should be attempted wherever possible. Having a 'placebo', that is something that looks like the treatment but is in fact inactive, makes it easier to blind a study. The theory and practice of RCTs developed in the very medical context of drug therapy. In this case, it is easy to make a pill that looks like the new drug but isn't. It has taken a long while for many surgical procedures to be subjected to the same rigorous assessment, partly because it is so difficult to blind the patient as to whether they have been operated on or not. However, there have been attempts to compare traditional surgery with keyhole surgery for a particular procedure, giving both groups of patients the same dressings. The fact that blinding has been attempted in such unlikely circumstances demonstrates the importance of blinding to the validity of an RCT. The issue of blinding becomes harder when you are comparing two quite different approaches to alleviate a condition. Depression may be treated with antidepressants. We might want to know whether alternatives, such as free gym sessions on prescription, or cognitive behaviour therapy, work just as well or better. In a trial that compared these approaches, it would be obvious to the participant which of these alternatives they were receiving. This applies to many Public Health interventions, making blinded RCTs of non-medical interventions difficult.

There are other challenges with conducting trials on Public Health interventions. Imagine you were interested in increasing levels of physical activity amongst teenage girls, and had identified a dance programme as an intervention to be tested.

Delivering this intervention through a school would seem a good way to reach the population of interest. If you randomised a sample of girls in the school to be offered extra dance sessions or not, you would find that some girls within each class were in the intervention group, while others were not. Some girls within particular friendship groups would be in the intervention group, while others would not. As well as being logistically challenging to organise, you may get a certain amount of 'contamination'. That is, girls receiving the intervention may influence their peers not receiving the intervention, so that the intervention increases physical activity levels in both the intervention and control group. One solution is to randomise groups of participants (classes or schools in this case) rather than individuals. This approach is commonly used in Public Health, and often makes the organisation of trials simpler. The unit of randomisation may be school, clinic, GP surgery, or nursing home, for example. A recent trial randomised wards within a hospital to a smoking cessation intervention, compared with usual practice (Murray et al. 2013). It would have been harder logistically to give individual patients on the same ward different smoking cessation services. This example also illustrates one of the problems with cluster randomisation—randomisation resulted in the wards in the two arms of the trial being quite different in terms of specialty and patient characteristics. This is a particular problem if the number of clusters to be randomised is small.

> **Discussion Task**
> Is an experimental study design always superior to an observational study design?

Systematic Review

A systematic review provides an overview of primary research to answer a particular research question. The aim is to identify, select, synthesise and appraise all high quality research evidence relevant to answering the question. Reviews on particular topics have long been published by experts in the field, but these are prone to selective reporting and bias. The key thing about a systematic review is that it minimises bias by using explicit, systematic methods. This approach was championed by Archie Cochrane (2009). Cochrane reviews (http://www.cochranelibrary.com/) are internationally recognised as the highest quality systematic reviews to support evidence-based healthcare. Access to a reliable review of the current evidence to answer a particular research question becomes increasingly important as the amount of information available increases—it is very difficult for any professional to keep up with all the individual reports published in their field.

A systematic review starts with a clearly defined question. The next step is to identify all relevant research. This requires an appropriate search strategy and knowing the right databases for the topic. The search strategy should be transparent and reproducible. It is also important to search for unpublished research, through

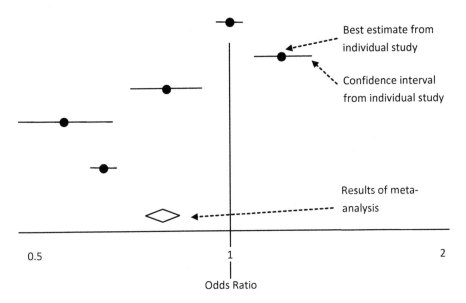

Fig. 8 Forest plot showing results of a systematic review

trial registers, for example. From the studies identified by the search strategy, those that are actually relevant to answering the question of interest need to be selected. Once those that should be included in the review have been agreed on, then each should be quality assessed (using a critical appraisal checklist or the Cochrane Risk of Bias Tool, for example). Studies of lower quality may be excluded at this stage. The next stage is to extract the results from each paper, using a standardised form to ensure consistency. Finally, the results of the individual studies can be compared. If the studies are sufficiently similar to one another (heterogeneous) in terms of the exact intervention delivered, the population of interest, and the follow-up time, then it may be appropriate to combine the results of the various studies.

This statistical analysis is called a meta-analysis. Essentially, it averages the results across studies, weighting by the size of the study. If a meta-analysis is performed, then the overall results are shown by a diamond at the bottom (see Fig. 8). In this graph, each black circle represents an individual study, and the horizontal lines through each show the confidence intervals. Sometimes, the studies are shown by squares proportional to the size of the study, and it is clear that larger studies tend to have narrower confidence intervals. The width of the diamond denotes the confidence interval around the overall result. This demonstrates one of the major advantages of a systematic review—combining several small studies with relatively wide confidence intervals can result in an overall estimate that is considerably more precise and therefore much more useful for informing practice.

One of the major disadvantages of a systematic review is the problem of 'publication bias'. This arises because the direction and statistical significance of research results will affect the likelihood of it getting published. This form of bias starts with the researchers themselves, who are less likely to write up and submit for publication the results of a study if it does not show something new and interesting. It extends to journal reviewers, who are likely to be more impressed by significant findings regardless of the study quality, and to journal editors who want to carry exciting research 'stories', much like newspaper editors. This is a serious problem when we try to combine all the evidence on one subject. We might find six studies saying that music therapy reduces severe depression, but what if there were another six studies which found no benefit at all (or even a negative effect), and these were not published? Then, our systematic review would draw a very erroneous conclusion. One way of testing for the existence of publication bias in a review is to plot the results of the various studies in what is called a 'funnel plot'. This identifies whether there appear to be any studies missing from the general pattern of results, but this approach only works when there are a good number of studies under consideration. A thorough search of the 'grey literature'—that is research not published in the peer-reviewed literature—is the best way to minimise publication bias. This might involve looking for Ph.D. theses and conference proceedings, internal reports of relevant organisations and talking to experts in the field.

Discussion Task
How can systematic reviews contribute to Public Health Intelligence?

Which Is the Most Appropriate Study Design?

An awareness of the hierarchy of evidence is useful for judging the reliability of research evidence. And while it is usually preferable to seek out a systematic review of all available evidence to answer a particular question, rather than relying on a single study, we cannot say that an RCT is always the best study design to use. It is more helpful to think about different study designs suiting different situations. Consider the following questions pertaining to tobacco smoking. If you wanted to answer the question 'What is the prevalence of smoking in this population, and how does it differ according to ethnicity?', then a cross-sectional study would be the most appropriate way to address this question. If you wanted to know how life-long smoking affects the risk of coronary heart disease and cancer, then a cohort study would enable you to answer this. But if the question was 'What is the most effective treatment to quit smoking?', then an RCT comparing various treatments would give the best quality evidence to answer this question. Finally, going beyond the traditional epidemiology discussed in this chapter, if you wanted to know why people continue to smoke, even when it is known to be harmful to health, then a qualitative approach would be best (i.e. talking to people to understand their decisions). Decisions about the most appropriate study design, therefore, depend upon an appreciation of the advantages and disadvantages of each (see Fig. 9).

Study Design	Advantages	Disadvantages
Case series	Quick, based on existing case notes	No control group, hypothesis generating only
Ecological study	Uses existing data sources	Depends on quality of data, ecological fallacy
Cross-sectional study	Good for descriptive statistics e.g. prevalence. Can collect data on a range of exposures and outcomes	Exposure and outcome measured at the same point in time Bias associated with poor response rates
Case-control study	Good for rare outcomes Can investigate multiple exposures Can be quick (e.g outbreak investigation)	Not good for rare exposures Recall bias Appropriate selection of controls Cannot estimate incidence
Cohort study	Good for measuring incidence Exposure measured before outcome. Can collect data on a range of exposures and outcomes Can investigate rare exposures if sample selected accordingly	Takes longer to collect data Drop-out over time leads to bias Difficult to control for confounding
Randomised Controlled Trial	Controls for confounding through randomisation Can collect data on multiple outcomes	Takes longer to collect data Can only compare 2 (or sometimes 3) interventions
Systematic review	Provides a summary of all available evidence Systematically addresses quality of individual studies	Prone to publication bias There may be heterogeneity between studies (in terms of population, intervention and

Fig. 9 Advantages and disadvantages of different study designs

Ethical Issues

A key ethical issue with all research designs involving primary data collection from human participants is consent. All participants should give consent to participate before they enter the study, in full knowledge of what this involves and understanding that they have the right to withdraw from the study at any point. There should be no coercion or pressure to take part. There are procedures in place for parents or guardians to give consent for children. Consent is also required to gain data on study participants through data linkage. When it comes to using anonymised secondary data, then access to the data will depend what purpose the data was collected for in the first place, and what consents if any have been obtained already for its use.

The sample size should be large enough to detect a difference or association if one really exists; otherwise, it is a waste of resources and unfair to the participants who are contributing to a study that has not been properly designed. Sample size calculations must take into account likely response rates and anticipated dropout over the course of follow-up. Studies should however not normally include more participants than is necessary, particularly if the research in invasive or particularly onerous for the participants.

Expenses incurred through being part of a study (e.g. travel) should be reimbursed. Participants may also be recompensed for their time, but incentives to take part are generally thought to be more problematic ethically. Nevertheless, the use of incentives can be very effective in improving response rates (Edwards et al. 2009), and might be approved by ethics committees when weighing up the benefits of achieving an adequate sample size.

Another ethical issue is what should be done if, during the course of a research study, a serious health condition or a high level of risk is discovered (e.g. dangerous drinking behaviour or suicidal thoughts). Protocols to deal with this situation must be agreed in advance. Although it is good practice to feed back the overall results of the study to participants, researchers need to decide whether to feed back any of the individual results. Participants of large cohort studies in the United States, for example, are often incentivised to take part by what they see as 'free health checks', whereas this type of individual feedback is less common in similar studies in the UK. Any potentially harmful effects of the research on the participants must be considered. These may be physical or mental. If asking questions about deliberate self-harm or drug misuse for example, it would be good practice to signpost relevant sources of help and information, and even to include a hotline number.

A key ethical issue in RCTs is whether it is appropriate to randomise at all. Although to epidemiologists the reasons for randomising are clear and we think of this as being the only sure way to test an intervention, it is much harder to convince the general public and even other professionals that randomising patients to receive a treatment or not is a good idea. There is a fear that this will lead to an apparent 'postcode lottery' with some people in an area receiving an intervention and others not. (One way round this problem is to use a cluster RCT, as described above.) An RCT is appropriate when there is what we call 'clinical equipoise'. That means that we genuinely don't know whether the new treatment to be tested is more (cost-)

effective than the standard treatment or, more generally, whether the intervention works. This applies whether we are talking about a new drug to treat cancer or a social policy intervention such as offering free nursery places to preschool children, or free school meals to all school children. Although there has traditionally been more acceptance of carrying out RCTs for medical interventions, and they are generally easier to organise than randomised trials of social interventions (which tend to be more complex and evolving), there is a growing trend to assess the effectiveness of policy decisions through the same rigorous approach as has long been applied to medicine.

> **Discussion Task**
> Explore some general ethical issues related to the design and conduct of epidemiological studies.

The Relevance of Epidemiology to Public Health Intelligence Today

Epidemiological information is used to investigate patterns of ill-health, generate and test hypotheses for the causes of ill-health, take action to prevent illness and promote health, and finally to evaluate existing health services and Public Health interventions. The role of epidemiology in Public Health practice is further discussed by Brownson (2011, p. 1).

The following examples of recent public heath news stories illustrate the application of epidemiology in practice: (1) an inner-city neighbourhood's concern about the rise in the number of children with asthma (*patterns of ill-health*), (2) findings published in a leading medical journal of an association between workers exposed to a chemical agent and an increased risk of cancer (*testing hypotheses*), (3) the revised recommendations for who should receive influenza vaccinations (*action to prevent illness*), and (4) the extensive disease-monitoring strategies being implemented in a city recently affected by a massive hurricane (*to enable evaluation of the disaster response*). In each case, the story relies on analysis and collation of Public Health intelligence. Identifying relevant data of the highest possible quality, understanding its limitations and interpreting it as useful information to help with Public Health planning and decision-making is the remit of Public Health Intelligence. London Health Observatory (2006) considers Public Health intelligence as 'The use of population information which has been analysed, interpreted and presented in clear and accessible form to inform proposed improvements to health services or to those factors which determine health, and which allow later examination to assess success'. This role has gained increasing importance with the shift towards evidence-based practice in Public Health (Killoran and Kelly 2009) which has followed the evidence-based medicine movement (Sackett et al. 1996).

Another recent trend is the need to include economic evaluations of Public Health interventions and health services, as well as evaluations of their efficacy and effectiveness. Public Health Economics is an area in which the Public Health workforce requires further training and capacity development. It includes techniques such as Social Return on Investment, which aims to capture all costs and benefits to society of a particular course of action, rather than those which are immediate, direct and easy to measure.

Many Public Health interventions are complex, spanning both health and social care and the anticipated benefits to society are often long term. In a climate of limited resources with a perpetual threat of funding cuts, the ability to capture data to accurately measure the return on investment in this way is clearly a priority for Public Health teams.

Discussion Task
Why is epidemiology the foundation and core principle of Public Health and Public Health intelligence?

Conclusion

Epidemiology is the cornerstone of Public Health. It employs rigorous methods and a quantitative approach to study the health of populations rather than individuals. Epidemiological methods are used to identify the causes of poor health, measure the strength of association between risk factors and disease, and evaluate interventions and monitor changes in population health over time. In short, epidemiology provides the necessary information for Public Health actions and decisions to be taken (see Carneiro and Howard 2011).

The main epidemiological study designs have been described, along with their strengths and limitations. In Public Health, interventions are often complex, and the exposures of interest are often known to be harmful in some way, or difficult to randomise for some other reason. In this situation, it is sometimes possible to conduct a natural experiment, but very often we have to rely heavily on observational study designs. Given that these are prone to bias and confounding, a pragmatic approach to identifying and quantifying likely biases is advisable. For a warning about the scale and implications of these biases, one needs only look at the contrasting evidence from cohort studies and randomised controlled studies on topics such as vitamin supplementation (Hooper et al. 2001; Egger et al. 2008).

Although the nature of epidemiology is changing, the key concept—that of assessing associations between potential risk factors and diseases or other health outcomes—remains the same. Developments in computing power make it ever more easy to model these relationships statistically, controlling for confounding, and assess the role of chance. The challenges of myriad forms of bias, and residual confounding, and the critical question of whether a relationship is causal are still very current.

References

Boyd, A., Golding, J., Macleod, J., Lawlor, D. A., Fraser, A., Henderson, J., et al. (2013). Cohort profile: The 'children of the 90s'—The index offspring of the Avon Longitudinal Study of Parents and Children. *International Journal of Epidemiology, 42*(1), 111–127.
Brownson, R. C. (2011). Epidemiology in Public Health practice [review of the book, by Haveman-Nies, A., Jansen, S., van Oers, H. and van 't Veer, P.]. *American Journal of Epidemiology, 174*(7), 871–872.
Carey, N. (2012). *The epigenetics revolution: How modern biology is rewriting our understanding of genetics, disease and inheritance.* London: Icon Books Ltd.
Carneiro, I., & Howard, N. (2011). *Introduction to epidemiology.* Maidenhead, England: McGraw-Hill Education.
Cochrane, A. L. (2009). *One man's medicine: An autobiography of Professor Archie Cochrane* (2nd ed.). Cardiff, England: Cardiff University.
Dyrstad, S. M., Hansen, B. H., Holme, I. M., & Anderssen, S. A. (2013). Comparison of self-reported versus accelerometer-measured physical activity. *Medicine and Science in Sports and Exercise, 46*(1), 99–106.
Edwards, P. J., Roberts, I., Clarke, M. J., Diguiseppi, C., Wentz, R., Kwan, I., et al. (2009). Methods to increase response to postal and electronic questionnaires. *Cochrane Database of Systematic Reviews, 8*(3), MR000008.
Egger, M., Davey, S. G., & Altman, D. G. (2008). *Systematic reviews in health care: Meta-analysis in context* (2nd ed.). London: Wiley-Blackwell.
Farr, W. (1974). Report on the mortality of cholera in England, 1848-9. In H. Ratcliffe (Ed.), Mortality in 19th century Britain. London: Gregg. Retrieved September 9, 2015, from http://johnsnow.matrix.msu.edu/work.php?id=15-78-12A
Hallquist, A., & Jansson, P. (2005). Self-reported diagnostic X-ray investigation and data from medical records in case-control studies on thyroid cancer: Evidence of recall bias? *European Journal of Cancer Prevention, 14*(3), 271–276.
Hooper, L., Ness, A. R., & Davey Smith, G. (2001). Meta-analysis of effect of high vs low vitamin E intake on cardiovascular mortality for observational and intervention studies (letter). *Lancet, 357*, 1705.
Killoran, A., & Kelly, M. P. (2009). *Evidence-based Public Health: Effectiveness and efficiency.* Oxford, England: Oxford University Press.
Last, J. M. (2001). *A dictionary of epidemiology* (4th ed.). Oxford, England: Oxford University Press.
London Health Observatory. (2006). Summary-mapping health intelligence in London. Retrieved August 24, 2015, from http://www.lho.org.uk/viewResource.aspx?id=10898
Madsen, K. M., Hviid, A., Vestergaard, M., Schendel, D., Wohlfahrt, J., Thorsen, P., et al. (2002). A population-based study of measles, mumps, and rubella vaccination and autism. *New England Journal of Medicine, 347*(19), 1477–1482.
McBride, W. G. (1961). Thalidomide and congenital abnormalities. *Lancet, 2*, 1358.
Murray, R. L., Leonardi-Bee, J., Marsh, J., Jayes, L., Li, J., Parrott, S., et al. (2013). Systematic identification and treatment of smokers by hospital based cessation practitioners in a secondary care setting: Cluster randomised controlled trial. *British Medical Journal, 347*, f4004.
Sackett, D. L., Rosenberg, W. M. C., Gray, J. A. M., Haynes, R. B., & Richardson, W. S. (1996). Evidence-based medicine: What it is and what it isn't. *British Medical Journal, 312*, 71–72.
Snow, J. (1855). *On the mode of communication of cholera* (2nd ed.). London: Churchill.
Tannous, L. K., Barlow, G., & Metcalfe, N. H. (2014). A short clinical review of vaccination against measles. *Journal of Royal Society of Medicine Open, 5*(4), 1–6.
Wakefield, A. J., Murch, S. H., Anthony, A., Linnell, J., Casson, D. M., Malik, M., et al. (1998). Ileal-lymphoid-nodular hyperplasia, non-specific colitis and pervasive developmental disorder in children. *Lancet, 35*, 637–641.
Wilkinson, R. G., & Pickett, K. (2010). *The spirit level: Why equality is better for everyone* (2nd ed.). London: Penguin Books.

Recommended Reading

Bhopal, R. (2008). *Concepts of epidemiology* (2nd ed.). Oxford, England: Oxford University Press.

Bonita, R., Beaglehole, R., & Kjellström, T. (2006). *Basic epidemiology* (2nd ed.). Geneva, Switzerland: World Health Organization.

Centre for Disease Control and Prevention. (2006). *An introduction to applied epidemiology and biostatistics*. Atlanta, GA: CDC.

Gordis, L. (2014). *Epidemiology* (5th ed.). Oxford, England: Elsevier Saunders.

Types of Data and Measures of Disease

Jacqui Dorman and Ivan Gee

Abstract Public health intelligence is the ongoing systematic collection, analysis, interpretation, and dissemination of health and social care data. Public health professionals use data to describe and monitor health-related events in their areas (local, regional, and national). Analysis of this information allows for effective setting of public health priorities, planning, implementation, and ultimately evaluation of public health interventions, programmes, and services. This chapter aims to describe the key data sources accessed and the different statistical methods and techniques, used to determine the burden of disease in populations and where these populations may be geographically or demographically placed.

By the end of this chapter, you should be able to:

• Understand the data sources used in public health
• Understand the different measures of disease used in public health
• Understand how to interpret measures of disease
• Understand the basic principles of data quality and information governance

Part I: Understanding Data Sources

The purpose of public health intelligence is to monitor the patterns of disease occurrence and the factors that might lead to poor public health within a population so that we can be effective in investigating, controlling, and preventing disease in that population and ensuring that the relevant interventions and services are placed where they will be most effective. To do this active engagement with a wide variety of data sources is required.

J. Dorman (✉)
Public Health, Tameside MBC, 19 Course View, Oldham OL4 5QB, UK
e-mail: jacqui.dorman@tameside.gov.uk

I. Gee
Center for Public Health, Liverpool John Moores University,
Henry Cotton Building, 15–21 Webster St, Liverpool L3 2ET, UK

© Springer International Publishing Switzerland 2016   41
K. Regmi, I. Gee (eds.), *Public Health Intelligence*,
DOI 10.1007/978-3-319-28326-5_3

Data sources used predominately in public health comprise:

- Demographic data sets
- Hospital activity data sets
- Birth data sets, death data sets
- Health and social care data sets

These are generally available at pseudonymised level (not patient identifiable). With the exception of births and mortality data, these data sets do allow access to postcode, which allows analysts to explore how health varies geographically across an area.

The health and social care system produces vast amounts of data daily, which, if used effectively, can be transformed into intelligence that will inform the commissioning decisions for health and social care organisations, help improve population health and well-being, improve clinical journeys for service users, and identify health inequalities.

The following sections will briefly explore important data sources.

Discussion Task
What is data and why do you need to know about data?

Comment: This is perhaps summed up well by Pencheon (2006), 'Some people are purists. They use the word 'data' (singular or plural) for raw numbers or other measures, reserving the word 'information' for what emerges when data are processed, analysed, interpreted, and presented. This has the virtue of making clear the sequence of steps that are involved in turning observations about the world into a form that is useful to those who wish to draw conclusions, and to act' (p. 80).

Public Health Birth files

The registration of births and deaths in the UK is a service delivered by:

(a) The Local Registration Service in England and Wales in partnership with the General Register Office (GRO). Since 1 April 2008, GRO has been part of the Identity and Passport Service.
(b) National Records of Scotland (NRS).
(c) General Register Office for Northern Ireland (GRONI)

Life event statistics for England and Wales are provided by the Office for National Statistics. Data for Scotland are provided by National Records Scotland and Northern Ireland's are produced by the Northern Ireland Statistics and Research Agency. Overall statistics for the UK are compiled by the Office for National Statistics.

Quarterly birth statistics for the UK and its constituent countries are based on the details collected when births are registered. "Provisional birth statistics" for the first three quarters of each year are published around 5 months after the quarter has ended. Figures for the fourth quarter are published once quality assurance of the annual data set has been completed and final annual figures have been published and figures for the first three quarters are finalised. Provisional quarterly figures for births provide a timely indication of trends (ONS 2015). To receive quarterly birth statistics, receiver organisations need to have reached level 2 of the National Health Service (NHS) Information Governance (IG) toolkit.

> The Information Governance (IG) Toolkit is an online system which allows NHS organisations and partners to assess themselves against Department of Health IG policies and standards. It also allows members of the public to view participating organisations' IG Toolkit assessments. (*See below for further discussion about information governance*).

The data within the quarterly extract is used to calculate:

- Birth rates
- Fertility rates
- Conception rates
- Births by geographical residents
- Births by deprivation quintiles
- Births by residence of mother
- Births by age of mother
- Birth characteristics including low birth weight

Primary Care Mortality Database

The Primary Care Mortality Database (PCMD) holds mortality data as provided at the time of registration of the death along with additional GP details, geographical indexing and coroner details where applicable.

Currently, the database contains data from 2006 and is based on the 2011 census structures. Monthly data is added by the second week of the following month.

User access to the data is based on the Upper Tier Local Authority (LA) or Clinical Commissioning Group (CCG) structures that they are responsible for (HSCIC 2015a).

The data within the PCMD is used to calculate mortality rates such as <75 cancer mortality and All Age All-Cause Mortality (AAACM). It is used to monitor trends in mortality by different conditions, geographic area, demographic characteristics, and GP practice. Data is also used to calculate life expectancy, potential years of life lost, and excess winter mortality.

The PCMD is managed by the Health and Social Care Information Centre (HSCIC). Secure access is through Open Exeter via an N3 ('National Framework') connection.

PCMD data is supplied to users under:

(a) Section 42(4) of the Statistics and Registration Service Act (2007) (TSO 2007) as amended by section 287 of the Health and Social Care Act (2012)
(b) Regulation 3 of the Health Service (Control of Patient Information) Regulations 2002 (TSO 2002)

Information Governance and Data Security

Information Governance (IG) is a process that ensures necessary safeguards are in place to protect patient and personal information, while allowing for appropriate use. The principles of information security require that all reasonable care is taken to prevent inappropriate access, modification, or manipulation of data from taking place.

In practice, this is applied through three cornerstones—**confidentiality, integrity, and availability** (HSCIC 2015b);

- **Confidentiality**: information must be secured against unauthorised access
- **Integrity**: information must be safeguarded against unauthorised modification
- **Availability**: information must be accessible to authorised users when they require it.

Data Security

To access the Primary Care Mortality Database, receiver organisations need to have reached level 2 of the NHS Information Governance toolkit.

'Even where access is granted, sharing of Patient Confidential Data obtained from PCMD, or the ONS files, cannot be passed to any other organisation, including the NHS, unless that organisation will also be using it for public health statistical purposes and has signed a Data Access Agreement for their organisation' (HSCIC 2015a, b, c, d, e, f).

For more information, see the HSCIC website: http://systems.hscic.gov.uk/infogov/codes

Secondary User Statistics

The Secondary Uses Service (SUS) is a single, comprehensive repository for health-care data in England which enables a range of reporting and analyses to support the organisations in the delivery of health care and public health services. SUS is a data repository for patient-level information that is held in a secure server and provides patient confidentiality to UK national standards. Data can be clear (patient identifiable), anonymised, or pseudonymised as required for the user's needs and their information governance accreditation (HSCIC 2015c).

SUS provides a range of information and tools which can be used to analyse and present data, SUS data. To access SUS data, an N3 connection ('National Framework') is required and attainment of NHS Information Governance toolkit level 2.

The SUS data warehouse contains data on admitted patient's care, outpatients, accident, and emergency statistics and can be used in practice for:

- Healthcare planning
- Commissioning services
- Payment by results
- Improving public health
- Developing national policy

Data from SUS can be used to monitor rates of hospital admissions from a wide range of conditions such as alcohol, self-harm, and mental health conditions. Hospital admissions can be used to gain an understanding into the burden of disease across different conditions, geographies, and communities. It is also used to monitor patient outcomes such as readmission rates and rates of hospital acquired infections.

Hospital Episode Statistics

Hospital Episode Statistics (HES) is a data warehouse containing details of all admissions, outpatient, appointments, and A&E attendances at NHS hospitals in England. The data is collected during a patient's time at hospital and is submitted to allow hospitals to be paid for the care they deliver.

HES data is designed to enable secondary use for non-clinical purposes such as public health provision. It is a records-based system that includes all NHS trusts in England (acute hospitals, CCGs, and mental health trusts). HES information is stored based on individual periods of care rather than patient by patient in a secure data warehouse (HSCIC 2015d).

Each HES record contains a range of information about an individual's admission, including:

- Clinical information about diagnoses and operations
- Information about the patient, such as age group, gender, and ethnicity

- Administrative information, such as time waited, and dates of admission and discharge
- Geographical information, such as where patients are treated and the area where they live

It contains data on admissions (from 1989), outpatient attendance data (from 2003), and A&E data (from 2007) (HSCIC 2015d). HES is a good alternative if access to Secondary User Statistics (SUS) data is not possible:
The purpose of HES is to (HSCIC 2015d):

- Monitor trends and patterns in NHS hospital activity
- Assess effective delivery of care
- Support local service planning
- Provide the basis for national indicators of clinical quality
- Reveal health trends over time
- Inform patient choice
- Determine fair access to health care
- Develop, monitor, and evaluate government policy
- Support NHS and parliamentary accountability

Vital Statistics

Vital statistics provide annual data for key statistics concerning: births, deaths, marriages, divorces, civil partnerships, and civil partnership dissolutions.

The purpose of the Vital Statistics data for England and Wales is to record numbers of conceptions, live births, stillbirths, deaths, and causes of death for England and Wales, according to gender and age group. Data are available from 1981, at various geographical levels: local authority, health authority, and ward. There have been changes over time to the recording of this data by the Office for National Statistics (ONS), which has resulted in some variations in the later content (UK Data Service 2015a).

Data can be provided to contacts in the NHS, Department of Health, NHS England and to Local Authorities (Public Health Analysts), providing they have signed the relevant ONS data access agreement. Vital statistics data is subject to disclosure control, which means that ONS will suppress any data that may identify an individual.

Disease Prevalence Data Sets

The Quality and Outcomes Framework (QOF) is a UK system for monitoring general practitioner (GP), activity, and performance and was introduced in 2004.

QOF awards surgeries achievement points for (HSCIC 2015e):

- Managing some of the most common chronic diseases, e.g. asthma, diabetes
- Implementing preventative measures, e.g. regular blood pressure checks
- The extra services offered such as child health care and maternity services
- The quality and productivity of the service, including the avoidance of emergency admissions to hospital
- Compliance with the minimum time a GP should spend with a patient at each appointment

Data on the prevalence of particular diseases or conditions is an important part of the Quality Outcomes Framework (QOF). Such data are used to calculate points and hence payments within clinical areas, but the data can have many other applications for public health intelligence.

QOF data is only collected at GP practice level so there is no centrally held information about individual patients that could be linked to the prevalence registers. This means that QOF data cannot be analysed by patient demographics such as age, gender, or socio-economic factors (DHSSPS, Northern Ireland 2015).

QOF data is only collected centrally at practice level. There is no centrally held data on patient details that can be directly linked to the prevalence data, so QOF data cannot be analysed by patient characteristics such as age or gender. The lack of patient-level data also prevents any analysis of comorbidity (patients being diagnosed with more than one condition). For example, information is collected for each GP practice on patients with coronary heart disease and separately for those patients with COPD, but QOF data does not show which patients have both COPD and heart disease (DHSSPS, Northern Ireland 2015).

QOF data is open access via the HSCIC website. It is generally published annually, a year in arrears.

National Data Sets

Public Health England

Public Health Observatories work jointly to generate information, data and intelligence on people's health and health care for health practitioners, policy makers, and society in general. They work toward national single work programmes to produce information on the following topic areas:

- General Health profiles
- Topic-based health profiles (tobacco, cancer, etc.)
- Data and knowledge gateway
- Screening
- Health inequalities
- Immunisation data and intelligence
- Small area indicators

For full details of data and intelligence resources produced by public health go to the Public Health England (PHE) website for more details of the tools and data resources they provide.

Census and ONS Population Data Sets

Census data and Office of National statistics population data sets enable public health to gain an understanding into the population and geodemographic characteristics of communities. Census and population data are accessed via the Office of National Statistics website.

The population census is an important resource for the development of public health research and policy development. It provides a snapshot of demographic and social life in the UK once every 10 years that can inform policy and practice (UK Data Service 2015b).

Population statistics derived from census data, such as mid-year population estimates, are used in the calculation of statistics such as hospital admission and mortality rates and life expectancy calculations. Population statistics are also used to ascertain the age and demographic breakdown of communities to enable commissioners to plan for future services that are age specific.

ImmForm

ImmForm is a website used by the Department of Health (DH), Public Health England (PHE), the National Health Service (NHS), and NHS England to:

- Collect data on vaccine uptake for immunisation programmes
- Collect data on incidence of influenza (flu) and influenza-like illness (ILI)
- Provide vaccine ordering facilities for the NHS
- Provide vaccination coverage information for secondary uses

The ImmForm website is used for the following vaccine uptake data collections in England:

- Seasonal flu (GP patients)
- Seasonal flu (prisons)
- Seasonal flu (frontline healthcare workers)
- HPV (human papillomavirus)
- Pertussis for pregnant women
- Shingles vaccine uptake
- Rotavirus vaccine uptake
- MMR catch up (GP Patients)
- PPV (pneumococcal polysaccharide vaccine)
- H1N1 ('swine flu') vaccine uptake

Uptake data for a number of childhood vaccinations are collected by PHE via the COVER (Cover of Vaccination Evaluated Rapidly) data collection. Uptake data for Td/IPV (school-leaving booster), MMR uptake in 13- to 18-year-olds and BCG are collected by the Information Centre on the KC50 return.

This data is used to monitor vaccination coverage at different age, gender, and geographic levels. It is used as part of the health protection element of the public health service locally.

NHS Indicator Portal

HSCIC provides an Indicator Portal which compiles a range of health indicators together in one website. It aims to provide quick and easy access to a large number of health-related indicators (HSCIC 2015f).

Data in the indicator portal includes:

- Compendium of Population Health Indicators
- Local Basket of Inequalities Indicators (LBOI)
- GP Practice data
- Social Care data
- The Adult Social Care Outcomes Framework
- Quality Accounts
- NHS Outcomes Framework
- Summary Hospital-level Mortality Indicator (SHMI)

The data on the portal can be used to (HSCIC 2015f):

- Compare the demographic profiles of different local areas and with national averages
- Identify public health issues in an area and their change over time
- Examine the range of factors that can influence health inequalities in an area
- Identify health inequalities in an area for health assessments and equity audits
- Provide information to inform service planning and performance

Discussion Task
Thinking about the area you live, go to the indicator portal https://indicators. ic.nhs.uk/webview/ and search for mortality from cardiovascular disease, DSR, <75 years, 3 year average, MFP; for where you live, the region you live and England.

How does your area compare? Discuss.

Cancer Commissioning Toolkit

The Cancer Commissioning Toolkit (CCT) was developed to support NHS Commissioners and Providers by providing suitable intelligence on cancer. The data can assist in identifying patterns of care and different service options that are effective and provide good value for money. It can also promote information sharing to help improve the patient experience. The toolkit provides population-level data sets, benchmarking, charting, and profiles (NCIN 2015). The main aim of the CCT is to provide data and intelligence around cancer in one place.

Examples of the information included in the toolkit include:

- Bowel, breast, and cervical screening
- Incidence
- Prevalence
- Routes to diagnosis
- Staging
- Recovery
- Survival
- Mortality
- Surgical procedures
- Expenditure

Part II: Measures of Disease

Public health intelligence measures the distribution, determinants, and burden of disease in populations. The objectives of public health intelligence are to determine the extent of disease in populations, identify patterns and trends, identify causes of disease, and evaluate the effectiveness of prevention and intervention. In order to use data effectively to achieve the above, various methodologies of disease measurements are used that transfer numbers into usable and comparable measures of disease.

Data Quality

High quality and reliable data is required for analysis and for accurately evaluating the impact of public health interventions and measuring public health outcomes. We need:

- Accurate and timely data to evaluate public health outcomes and services
- High quality information to evaluate service effectiveness and ensure value for money

Underlying data quality is fundamental to the values of any derived statistics produced. Data quality has a number of components:

- Completeness—refers to the available data fields needed to fulfil analytical requirements; it is defined as the percentage or number of data missing from a given dataset. For example, only date of birth fields being 65 % complete
- Accuracy—refers to data values within a given dataset, for example, date of birth given 23/5/1964 but age is given at 15 years when it should read 51 years
- Relevance—refers to the impact of specific data on the decision-making process, too little may not give the full picture of needs to much data can lead to 'information overload' and therefore complicate the decision-making process
- Timeliness—refers to the speed of dissemination of the data—i.e. the period between the end of a data set (or a reference date) and distribution of the data?

Data quality can also be checked by using the 'CART' acronym (Pencheon 2006):

C: completeness
A: accuracy
R: relevance (and or representative)
T: timeliness

Assessing data quality often begins when intelligence professionals discover that a particular database contains errors. Data quality procedures use a series of methods to improve data quality, including:

- Data profiling—examining the data to determine its overall accuracy
- Data standardisation—using predetermined criteria to ensure that the data matches defined quality levels
- Geocoding—automated matching tools to fix common errors, e.g. name and address data
- Matching and linking—comparing records to match similar but slightly different entries, e.g. the same persons details but recorded with and without their middle initial
- Monitoring—continual assessment of data quality

Discussion task
What are the fundamental issues which affect the quality of data and why is data quality important? Discuss.

The following sections describe the most commonly used public health measures.

Life Expectancy

Definition: the average number of years that a newborn is expected to live if current mortality rates continue to apply (WHO 2015).

Methodology: Life expectancy is calculated by constructing a life table which uses just the population of an area and the number of deaths in the area (or the age-specific death rates). Life expectancy figures are generally calculated as 3-year rolling averages to provide larger numbers which increases the robustness of the estimates (LHO 2015). For very small geographic areas, such as wards, 5 years worth of mortality data might be needed. Examples of life tables and a calculator can be found on the PHE website.

Interpretation: Life expectancy figures represent the typical mortality for people living in an area. For a specific area, it estimates the average number of years a newborn baby would live **if** they experienced the overall age-specific mortality rates for that area throughout their life. The figures don't tell us how many years a baby born in the area will actually expect to live. This is because the mortality rates for the area are likely to change over time and because many people will live elsewhere for some part of their lives (Public Health England 2015).

> **The Ecological Fallacy**
> We need to beware of applying statistics such as life expectancy that are based on population averages to individuals. Doing this is a common mistake, called the Ecological Fallacy. An individual's lifespan will be largely determined by factors that are specific to the individual such as lifestyle, family history, housing, and conditions. Applying population-based estimates to an individual does not account for these personal factors.

Healthy Life Expectancy

Definition: This is the average number of years a person would expect to live with good health based on mortality rates and the prevalence of self-reported good health (Public Health England 2015).

Methodology: Healthy life expectancy is calculated from abridged Sullivan life tables using 5 year age bands. Sullivan life tables extend normal life table calculations by dividing the years lived into favourable and unfavourable health states to estimate healthy life expectancy, based on surveys such as the Annual Population Survey that collect data on self-reported health. The calculations are performed separately for males and females (Public Health England 2015).

Interpretation: Healthy Life expectancy figures represent the prevalence of good health and mortality for people living in an area and. It estimates the average number of years a newborn baby would live in good general health **if** they experienced the area's age-specific mortality rates and prevalence of good health throughout their life.

Prevalence

Definition: The proportion of a population who have a disease at a point in time is the **'prevalence of disease'**. It is often expressed as a percentage. The 'point in time' can be a single examination (point prevalence), but is often a longer time scale in order to give a better estimate of the numbers with the disease (period prevalence). Prevalence is mainly used for diseases that are chronic, such as asthma, diabetes, cardiovascular disease, and chronic obstructive pulmonary disease (Dorman 2009).

Methodology: Prevalence is calculated by dividing the number of observed events of a health indicator during a specified time period (e.g. cases of diabetes) by the size of the population in which the health indicator occurs. The result is often expressed as a percentage.

$$\text{Prevalence} = \frac{\text{persons with a given health indicator during as pecified time period}}{\text{population during the same time period}} \times 100$$

Example

If 12,000 residents in a local authority with a total population of 160,000 residents have hypertension, the prevalence of hypertension in this local authority is calculated as:

$$\text{Prevalence of hypertension} = \frac{22,000}{160,000} \times 100$$

$$\text{Prevalence of hypertension} = 13.75\%$$

Incidence

Incidence is the rate at which new cases of a disease, condition, or behaviour occur in a specified population. It is usually reported as the number of new cases occurring over a set period of time (e.g. per year) as a fraction of the total population at risk of developing the disease (e.g. per 100,000 population) (Dorman 2009).

Methodology: The incidence is calculated by dividing the number of newly observed (or diagnosed) events by the total population risk multiplied by 100,000 (or other suitable multiplier).

$$\text{Incidence} = \frac{\text{persons with a new diagnosis of a given health indicator}}{\text{population a trisk}} \times 100,000$$

Example

If in a week in October, 149 students in a university halls of residents are treated for symptoms relating to food poisoning. During the same week, 5000 students ate lunch in the same restaurant as the students showing symptoms. The incidence of food poisoning among students during this week in October is calculated as:

$$\text{Incidence of food poisoning} = \frac{149}{5000} \times 100,000$$
$$\text{Incidence of food poisoning} = 2980 \text{ per } 100,000$$

The incidence in food poisoning in students is therefore 2980 per 100,000 people. This is a large number that is not that easy to present so depending on how common the problem is we can use alternative population multipliers to the 100,000 we used here. So for this example we could multiply by 1000 instead, so the Incidence of food poisoning would be 29.8 per 1,000.

$$\text{Incidence} = 2980 \text{ per } 100,000 \text{ people} = 29.8 \text{ per } 1000 \text{ population}$$

Interpretation: Incidence is useful for studying the changes in levels of disease and for examining the causes of disease. Incidence looks at the rate at which new events occur in a population while prevalence describes the total amount or extent of a disease, condition, or behaviour. While prevalence is affected by factors such as how long people live with a condition, effectiveness of treatments, remission, and relapse, incidence is not affected by these.

Figure 1 illustrates the difference between incidence and prevalence, imagining the population as a pool of water. Prevalence is the total number of cases within the pool, incidence is the number of new cases flowing into the pool, which increases prevalence. Mortality and remission (either natural or due to effective treatment) remove cases from the pool, so reduce prevalence.

Standardisation (Direct and Indirect)

Definition: The problem with the so-called crude rates like incidence and prevalence is that they are influenced by confounding factors that may vary between areas. For example, Southport has, on average, an older population than central Liverpool. Southport has many retirees; Liverpool has many students. As the population is older, we would expect Southport to have higher mortality and morbidity,

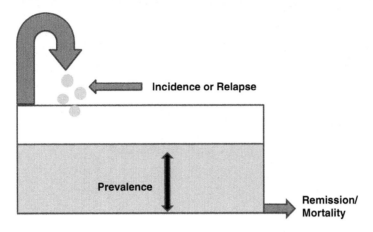

Fig. 1 The relationships between incidence, prevalence, remission, and mortality

just due to the confounder of age, older people tend to have more disease than younger people. Standardisation of rates tries to account for differences in the age of populations in different areas to allow 'fairer' comparisons in levels of disease. But accounting for the difference in age of different areas we can then see that there are other underlying differences in disease rates, which are not due to age but might be due to inequalities, different behaviours, more effective services, etc.

There are two methods of standardisation commonly used in public health: direct and indirect. Direct methods use a standard population distribution and indirect methods use a standard set of age-specific rates. Both methods involve the calculation of numbers of expected events in an area (e.g. deaths), which are compared to the actual number of observed events (Health Knowledge 2011).

Direct Standardisation

Directly standardised rates (DSRs) give an indication of the number of events that would occur in a standard population if that population had the same age-specific rates as the local area. The most commonly used standard population is the European Standard population; however, other populations such as the England, or World standard population can also be used. The rates are calculated per 100,000 and because rates are applied to the same population, rates across areas can be directly compared, hence direct standardisation (Dorman 2009).

Unlike indirect standardised rates, which compare the observed number of events to the expected number of events, DSRs can be used to compare disease rates directly across areas and time. DSRs are of particular use in assessing the relative burden of disease in a population, e.g. if there is more heart disease than cancer, and for directly comparing areas to identify where problems are more severe (Dorman 2009).

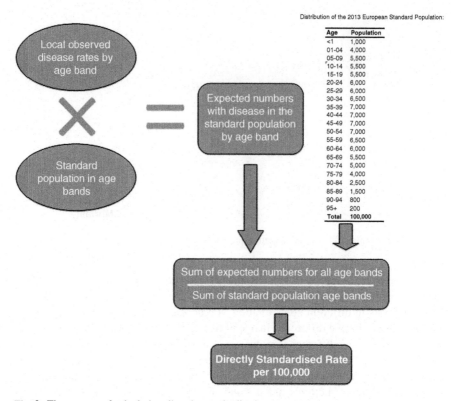

Distribution of the 2013 European Standard Population:

Age	Population
<1	1,000
01-04	4,000
05-09	5,500
10-14	5,500
15-19	5,500
20-24	6,000
25-29	6,000
30-34	6,500
35-39	7,000
40-44	7,000
45-49	7,000
50-54	7,000
55-59	6,500
60-64	6,000
65-69	5,500
70-74	5,000
75-79	4,000
80-84	2,500
85-89	1,500
90-94	800
95+	200
Total	100,000

Fig. 2 The process of calculating directly standardised rates

Methodology: A DSR is calculated by dividing the number of observed deaths/hospital admissions by age band (usually 5 year age bands) by the local population (also by age band) multiplied by the European Standard population (ESP). Once the calculation has been made across all age bands the DSR is then calculated by summing all the age bands together to give a total DSR outcome.

Figure 2 shows this process as a diagram.

$$\text{DSR} = \sum \frac{\text{condition counts (in 5 year age bands)}}{\text{population (in 5 year age bands)}} \times \text{ESP (in 5 year age bands)}$$

Interpretation: The aim of standardisation is to provide a summary 'adjusted' rate that takes into account underlying differences in the age structure of the study, or target, population relative to a 'reference' or standard population. Once calculated for different areas the DSRs are directly comparable with rates from other areas. Both have been calculated using the same reference population and hence have the same underlying age structure. Any differences between the rates can be attributed to factors other than age.

When you need to calculate a DSR for specific age groups rather than all ages in 5 year age bands (e.g. for 0–74 years, or age 55+), you can use the same methodology but calculate a 'truncated' rate. This is achieved by ignoring the data for the population above or below the specified age limits.

When the numbers of events are small (e.g. deaths from rare cancers), the calculated rates may be less reliable. The rule of thumb is not to use direct standardisation for numbers of events under 50. Standardisation may also be misleading in some cases because the standardised rate summarises the data into just one number, which can hide patterns in specific age groups or between the sexes. You should always look carefully at the data to try and understand the population before standardising (Finlayson et al. 2011).

Indirect Standardisation

Indirect standardisation compares the actual numbers of events (observed) in the local or target population to expected numbers calculated from a reference or standard population, adjusting for age and sex. This produces a ratio (observed/expected) that is commonly called a standardised mortality ratio, or an SMR. The expected number of deaths is calculated from the age-specific death rates from a larger reference population, such as the national population (Health Knowledge 2011).

Depending on the data used, indirect standardisation can produce the following measures (Finlayson et al. 2011):

- Standardised Mortality/Morbidity Ratio (SMR): when using mortality or morbidity data
- Standardised Incidence Ratio (SIR): when using disease incidence data
- Standardised Registration Ratio (SRR): when using registration data (e.g. for cancers)
- Standardised Operation Ratio (SOR): when using hospital operation data.

Methodology: The indirectly standardised ratio is calculated by dividing the observed number of events (deaths, hospital admissions, etc.) by the expected number, multiplied by 100. The expected number of events is calculated by applying the death rates (typically in 5 year age bands) for the reference population to the numbers of people in the study population (again in specified age bands) and then summing those expected age-specific events.

$$\text{Standardised Ratio} = \frac{\text{observed condition count}}{\text{expected count}} \times 100$$

As the Standard Ratio of the reference population is always 100 a value of lower than 100 means that for example in the case of deaths, **fewer deaths than expected** occurred in the local population after adjusting for differences in age and sex; a value greater than 100 means that there have been **more deaths than expected**.

Confidence Intervals

Definition: A confidence interval gives an estimated range of values which is likely to include an unknown population limitation, the estimated range being calculated from a given set of sample data (Dorman 2009).

If independent samples are taken repeatedly from the same population, and a confidence interval calculated for each sample, then a certain percentage (confidence level) of the intervals will include the unknown population limitation. Confidence intervals are usually calculated so that this percentage is 95 %, but we can produce 90, 99, and 99.9 % confidence intervals for the unknown limitation (Dorman 2009).

In public health many indicators are calculated from virtually complete data sets and not samples, e.g. mortality rates based on registered deaths. In these circumstances, the uncertainty about the indicator comes derives from 'natural' variation not the normal sampling variations. The indicator is result of a stochastic process (i.e. one which can be influenced by the random occurrences in the world around us). So the value observed from the data is only one of a set of values that could naturally occur. In public health, it is the underlying circumstances or process that is of interest so in these case the value of the observed indicator only provides an estimate of this 'underlying risk' (APHO 2008).

Methodology: Confidence interval calculations will be different depending on the outcome measure. We need different calculations for different types of data. The formula below is an example of a confidence interval formula which is used for calculating confidence intervals in rates and ratios.

The upper and lower confidence limits $100(1-\alpha)\%$, for the DSR are given by (APHO 2008):

$$\text{DSR}_{\text{lower}} = \text{DSR} + \sqrt{\frac{\text{Var}(\text{DSR})}{\text{Var}(O)}} \times (O_{\text{lower}} - O)$$

$$\text{DSR}_{\text{upper}} = \text{DSR} + \sqrt{\frac{\text{Var}(\text{DSR})}{\text{Var}(O)}} \times (O_{\text{upper}} - O)$$

where

O is the total observed count of events in the local or subject population
O_{lower} and O_{upper} are the lower and upper limits for the observed count of events
$\text{Var}(O)$ is the variance of the total observed count O
$\text{Var}(\text{DSR})$ is the variance of the DSR
α is the level of confidence required, e.g. 5 %.

Interpretation: To estimate the likelihood that a result is caused by something other than mere chance, the width of the confidence interval gives us some idea about how certain we are about the value of the health indicator. Wide intervals indicate we are not very confident of the true value of the indictor, a narrow interval indicates we have much greater confidence in its value. In general, narrower confidence intervals

No Overlap: Significantly different   Lots of Overlap: Not Significantly different

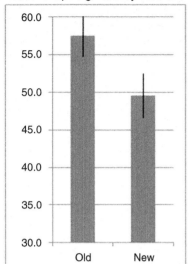   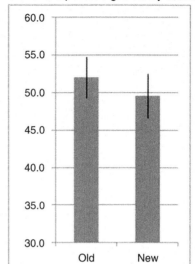

Fig. 3 Examples of significant and non-significant confidence intervals

will be obtained where we have used large data sets, if we have wide confidence intervals we might need more data before we can be very definite about the outcome.

Confidence intervals are a very effective way of making comparisons between two or more different estimates, for example, between different organisations, areas, or time periods. By comparing the confidence intervals of the estimates to see if they overlap, we can determine if there is a statistically significant difference between the two estimated values. Non-overlapping confidence intervals are considered to be statistically significantly different (APHO 2008) (Fig. 3).

Confidence intervals should be presented alongside the point estimate of the indicator wherever an inference is being made from a sample to a population or from a set of observations to the underlying process (or 'risk') that generated them (APHO 2008).

There are tools and templates available on the PHE website that will help with the calculation of common public health statistical indicators.

Years of Life Lost

Definition: Potential years of life lost (YLL) provide a summary measure of premature mortality. Potential years of life lost may be defined as the number of years of potential life lost due to early death. YLL takes into account the age at which deaths occur, giving greater weight to deaths at a younger age and lower weight to deaths at older age (Health Knowledge 2009).

YLL is used in public health intelligence to allow a comparison between the relative importance of different causes of premature deaths within a population of interest. This allows us to compare premature mortality between populations which might help identify areas of good practice that can be used in other areas, or areas with significant problems that can be prioritised for interventions (Health Knowledge 2009).

Methodology: The number of YLL is calculated by summing the number of deaths at each age between 1 and 74 years, and multiplying by the number of years of life remaining (up to the age of 75 years) (Health Knowledge 2009).

$$YLL = \sum_{74}^{i-1} a_i d_i$$

Where:

i = age
a_i = no. years of life remaining to age 75 when death occurs between ages i and $i+1$
d_i = no. observed deaths in the population between ages i and $i+1$

Assuming a uniform distribution of deaths within age groups, $a_i = 75 - (i+0.5)$ therefore (Health Knowledge 2009):

$$YLL = \sum_{74}^{i-1} (74.5 - i) d_i$$

Interpretation: Potential years of life lost (YLL) is an indicator of premature or early death. If dying before the age of 75 is considered premature, then a person dying at age 55 would have lost 20 years of potential life. An area's YLL value will be higher if mortality among children or younger people is high. Conditions such as birth defects, injuries, and infectious disease outbreaks are major contributors to YLL values, whereas chronic diseases that cause deaths among the elderly will have little effect on the YLL (AIHW 2015).

YLL is a measure that focuses on death rates. So other measures of average health status such as disability-adjusted life years (DALYs) and quality-adjusted life years (QALYs) are increasing in use as these provide information not only on the length of life, but on the quality of life (AIHW 2015).

Quality-Adjusted Life Years (QALY) and Disability-Adjusted Life Years

Definition: Average life expectancy has increased but are these extra life years spent in good health or with disability?

QALYs are a measure of the state of health of a person or group, in terms of length of life, but adjusted to reflect the quality of life. One QALY is equal to 1 year of life in good health.

DALYs are a measure of the impact of a disease or injury in terms of healthy years lost to disability.

Methodology: A QALY is the amount of time spent in a health state weighted by the utility score given to that health state. Lower utility sores represent less than good health and mean that more time will be spent in that state in order to generate a QALY. For example, it takes 1 year of good health (with a utility score of 1) to generate one QALY, whereas 1 year in a health state valued at 0.5 is equivalent to half a QALY. So a public health intervention that generates 4 additional years in a health state valued at 0.75 will generate one more QALY than compared to 4 additional years of life without the intervention in a health state valued at 0.5 (Phillips and Thompson 2009).

A DALY is the sum of years of life lost (YLL) and the years lived with disability (YLD). One DALY equals 1 year of healthy life lost (DALY = YLD + YLL). The YLD are the morbidity component of the DALY, and are related to the number of cases and the severity of the disease. The YLL are the mortality component of the DALY, and are related to the number of deaths and the average age of death (Phillips and Thompson 2009).

Interpretation: QALYs: The QALY is a widely used economic indicator, which allows a consistent approach to comparing the value of different public health interventions. A QALY can be used to indicate how a public health intervention will benefit a population by considering:

- Quantity of life (how long you live for)
- Quality of life (the quality of your remaining years of life)

The QALY combines both these factors into a single value for the health benefits of any public health intervention. QALYs provide a benchmark that we can use to compare the benefits that each intervention is likely to offer.

The value of the QALY itself cannot tell you if an intervention provides value for money, but it can contribute to this. If we combine the QALY for a new public health intervention with the cost of that intervention, we can generate a ratio: the cost per QALY. The cost per QALY shows the extra QALY the new intervention gives for a particular cost.

DALYs: DALYs measure the losses in a population due to disability and/or deaths. So conditions and behaviours that account for more DALYs will have a greater public health impact than those producing fewer DALYs. Similarly, public health interventions will be favourable if they reduce the number of DALYs. DALYs can either be presented in absolute terms giving an indication of the total burden to the population, or they can be presented in relative terms, e.g. as the number of DALYs per 1000 population. Use of relative figures allows us to directly compare the health burden for different areas or population groups.

Correlation Coefficient

Definition: The correlation coefficient is always a value between −1 and +1 that indicates whether two sets of data (such as levels of smoking and lung cancer in different local authority areas) are statistically related. The closer to +1 the more 'confident' we are of a positive linear correlation (as one value goes up the other also rises, e.g. where we see more smoking we also tend to see more lung cancer) and the closer to −1 the more confident we are of a negative linear correlation (as one set of numbers decreases the other set increases, e.g. in areas where income increases we tend to see less lung cancer). When the correlation coefficient is close to zero, there is no evidence of any relationship.

Methodology: There are two methods of testing relationships between data sets used in public health intelligence. The Pearson correlation coefficient is the most widely used and measures the strength of the linear relationship assuming the data sets are both normally distributed. When the data sets are not normally distributed or the relationship between them is not linear, it may be more appropriate to use the Spearman rank correlation method.

Interpretation: Confidence in a relationship is formally determined not just by the correlation coefficient but also by the number of pairs in your data (the size of the data sets). If there are very few pairs (small data sets), then the coefficient needs to be stronger (very close to 1 or −1) for it to be considered 'statistically significant', but if there are many pairs then a coefficient closer to 0 can still be considered 'highly significant'. Statistical software will generally allow the calculation of probability values (p values) which can indicate the statistical significance of the correlation coefficient. So correlations often have two outputs, the correlation coefficient (r) which indicates the strength of the relationship and the statistical significance (p) which indicates the probability of the coefficient just being due to chance alone.

Example

To understand the results of Pearson's correlation coefficient, it is important to understand what the results are telling us. When calculating the coefficient, the formula calculated will return a value of r; this always lies in the range of −1 to +1. If the results lie close to either end of this range, then the spread of the values on a scatter graph will be small, and therefore a strong correlation between the two variables exists.

A value of +1 indicates that a high value of one variable is always associated with a value of the other variable. For example, an r value of 0.95 between DSRs for hospital admissions and percentage ward level BME populations indicates that a high DSR will always be associated with high percentage BME populations. On the other hand, a value of −1 indicates that a higher value of one variable (DSRs) is always associated with a lower value of the other variable (BME).

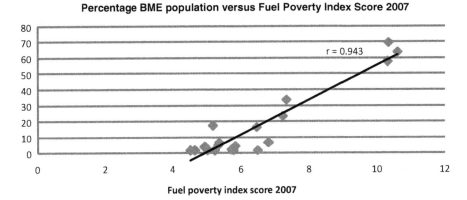

Fig. 4 Correlation between ward-level fuel poverty index scores and percentage BME

Figure 4 shows an example of a positive correlation between the % BME in different local areas and the fuel poverty scores for those areas. Using Pearson's correlation coefficient (r) and plotting data for ward level BME populations and fuel poverty on an XY scatter plot chart, along with a linear trend line. The chart illustrates that a strong, positive association exists between the fuel poverty index score and ward-level percentage BME population ($r = 0.94$).

r and r^2: There is often confusion between r (the correlation coefficient) and r^2 (the square of the correlation coefficient (also called the coefficient of determination). r values are produced from calculations of statistical correlations, r^2 values are produced by regression calculations of best fit lines. In the example from the graph, the Pearson's $r = 0.943$ so r^2 for the best fit line $= 0.89$ (i.e. 0.94×0.94).

> **Correlation and Confounding: Correlation Does Not Necessarily Mean Cause**
> The single most important thing to remember about correlations is that although correlation is an extremely valuable type of measure when used to look at cause and effect relationships between a treatment and benefit, or a risk factor and a disease, *correlation does not necessarily imply causality and must always be put into perspective*. For example, if we see a correlation between the amount of coffee people consume and the incidence of heart disease, this does not mean that coffee causes heart attacks. There may be some other factor (a confounding factor), such as stress, that causes people to drink more coffee, and causes the heart attacks.

Regression

Description: Regression is the process whereby two data sets are fitted to a linear best fit, regression line. The coefficient of determination (r^2) is a statistical measure of how closely the data match the fitted regression line and indicates how much of

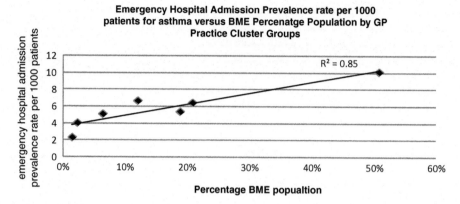

Fig. 5 Regression model indicating the extent that % BME can explain prevalence of asthma (estimated from hospital admissions)

the variation in one variable (dependent) can be explained by the other variable (independent).

r^2 is always between 0 and 1:

- 0 indicates that the regression model explains none of the variability in the dependent variable.
- 1.0 indicates that the model explains all the variability in the dependent variable

In general, the higher the r^2, the better the model fits your data. For example, looking at the chart below (Fig. 5), we can see that the r^2 is 0.85. This tells us that 85 % of the variability in emergency hospital admissions for asthma (r^2) is explained by percentage BME population with only 15 % of the variation being down to unexplained factors.

Conclusion

Public health intelligence is tasked with monitoring the health of populations and supporting interventions aimed at improving the health of the population. Public health intelligence uses statistical and epidemiological expertise to collate, analyse, and interpret data to support public health and the wider health and social care economy (Dorman et al. 2009). This chapter has covered the key data sources and common methodologies used in public health. It has touched on data quality and information governance and described the definition, methodologies, and interpretation of the most common statistical methodologies used in public health intelligence. The chapter has illustrated that public health intelligence uses many data sources and analytical techniques to identify the distribution and burden of disease in populations. However, there is a cross over between public health statistics, epidemiology, and medical statistics, and therefore if you require more in-depth knowledge, the following further reading is recommended.

References

AIHW. (2015). *Potential years of life lost.* Australian Institute of Health and Welfare. Retrieved September 30, 2015, from http://www.aihw.gov.au/WorkArea/DownloadAsset.aspx?id= 6442459114.

APHO. (2008). *Technical briefing 3: Commonly used public health statistics and their confidence intervals.* Association of Public Health Observatories. Retrieved September 30, 2015, from http://www.apho.org.uk/resource/view.aspx?RID=48457.

DHSSPS, Northern Ireland. (2015). *Factsheet—Prevalence data in the QOF.* Retrieved September 30, 2015, from www.dhsspsni.gov.uk/pd-qof-f.pdf.

Dorman, J. (2009). *Hospital admissions for asthma in Oldham: Are there any associations between characteristics of local GP practices and/or the wider determinants of health.*

Dorman, J., McCormack, A., & Carroll, P. (2009). *Public Health Intelligence e-Handbook: A guide for the public health analyst and wider workforce.* Retrieved September 23, 2015, from http:// s3.amazonaws.com/zanran_storage/www.gmphnetwork.org.uk/ContentPages/2481152558.pdf.

Finlayson, A., Springbett, A., & Burlison, A. (2011). *Calculation of standardised rates and ratios: Direct and indirect methods.* NHS Information Services Scotland. Retrieved September 30, 2015, from http://www.scotpho.org.uk/downloads/methodology/standardisation-guide-june-2011.doc.

Health Knowledge. (2011). *Standardisation.* Retrieved September 30, 2015, from http://www. healthknowledge.org.uk/e-learning/epidemiology/specialists/standardisation.

Health Knowledge. (2009). *Years of life lost.* Retrieved September 30, 2015, from http://www. healthknowledge.org.uk/public-health-textbook/research-methods/1a-epidemiology/ years-lost-life.

HSCIC. (2015a). *The primary care mortality database.* Retrieved September 30, 2015, from http:// www.hscic.gov.uk/pcmdatabase.

HSCIC. (2015b). *Principles of information security.* Retrieved September 30, 2015, from http:// systems.hscic.gov.uk/infogov/security.

HSCIC. (2015c). *Secondary uses service (SUS).* Retrieved September 30, 2015, from http://www. hscic.gov.uk/sus.

HSCIC. (2015d). *Hospital episode statistics.* Retrieved September 30, 2015, from http://www. hscic.gov.uk/hes.

HSCIC. (2015e). *Online GP practice results database.* Retrieved September 30, 2015, from http:// qof.hscic.gov.uk/0506/.

HSCIC. (2015f). *Indicator portal.* Retrieved September 30, 2015, from http://www.hscic.gov.uk/ indicatorportal.

London Health Observatory (LHO). (2015). *Calculating life expectancy and infant mortality rates.* Retrieved September 30, 2015, from www.lho.org.uk/download.aspx?urlid=7656.

NCIN. (2015). *Cancer commissioning toolkit (CCT).* Retrieved September 30, 2015, from http:// www.ncin.org.uk/cancer_information_tools/cct.

Office for National Statistics. (2015). *Live births and stillbirths.* Retrieved September 3, 2015, from http://www.ons.gov.uk/ons/taxonomy/index.html?nscl=Live+Births+and+Stillbirths.

Pencheon, D. (2006). *Using data and evidence*: Introduction. Oxford handbook of public health practice (2nd ed., p. 80). New York: Oxford University Press.

Phillips, C., & Thompson, G. (2009). *What is a QALY?* What is Series…? (2nd ed.) Publishers: Hayward Medical Communications. Retrieved September 30, 2015, from http://www.medicine.ox.ac.uk/bandolier/painres/download/whatis/qaly.pdf

Public Health England. (2015). *Public health outcomes framework.* Retrieved September 30, 2015, from http://www.phoutcomes.info/public-health-outcomes-framework#gid/1000049/ pat/6/ati/102/page/6/par/E12000004/are/E06000015.

The Stationery Office. (2007). *Statistics and Registration Service Act 2007* (Chapter 18). Retrieved September 3, 2015, from http://www.legislation.gov.uk/ukpga/2007/18/contents.

The Stationery Office. (2002). *The health service (control of patient information) regulations 2002.* Retrieved September 3, 2015, from http://www.legislation.gov.uk/uksi/2002/1438/schedules/made.
UK Data Service. (2015a). *Vital statistics for England and Wales.* Retrieved September 30, 2015, from https://discover.ukdataservice.ac.uk/series/?sn=2000055.
UK Data Service. (2015b). *About census support.* Retrieved September 30, 2015, from http://census.ukdataservice.ac.uk/about-us.
WHO. (2015). *Life expectancy at birth.* Retrieved September 30, 2015, from www.who.int/whosis/whostat2006DefinitionsAndMetadata.pdf.

Recommended Reading

Carneiro, I., & Howard, N. (2011). *Introduction to epidemiology: Understanding public health* (2nd ed.). Oxford, England: Oxford University Press.
Carr, S., Unwin, N., & Pless-Mulloli, T. (2007). *An introduction to public health epidemiology* (2nd ed.). Maidenhead, England: Open University Press.
Harris, M., & Taylor, G. (2014). *Medical statistics made easy* (3rd ed.). Banbury, England: Scion.
Stewart, A. (2010). *Basic statistics and epidemiology: A practical guide* (3rd ed.). Buckinghamshire, England: Radcliffe.
Webb, P., & Bain, C. (2010). *Essential epidemiology: An introduction for students and health professionals.* Cambridge, England: Cambridge University Press.

Modelling in Public Health

Adam Briggs, Peter Scarborough, and Adrian Smith

Abstract This chapter outlines the main uses and challenges of modelling in public health. Individual model methods are discussed alongside examples of their use. This will help you to interpret public health models and to be aware of some of their main assumptions, thereby allowing you to use models more appropriately in your day-to-day work.

After reading this chapter, you will be able to:

- Know when it is and is not appropriate to use modelling in public health.
- Be confident when using model outcomes in your day-to-day work.
- Be able to explain the common modelling methods to colleagues.
- Understand different modelling methods and their main strengths and limitations.

Introduction

Public health decision makers need to consider a wide range of options and outcomes when considering how best to approach an identified public health need. For example, what proportion of the population undergoing a new screening programme will benefit and what proportion will be harmed? What will happen to levels of obesity over the next 20 years? How many cases of influenza should we expect in the local nursing home population this year? Is putting in a new cycle route more cost-effective than a healthy food advertising campaign for reducing obesity?

Such questions are difficult, if not impossible, to answer using empirical research either because such research is very costly, is unethical to carry out, or would take too

A. Briggs (✉) • P. Scarborough • A. Smith
Nuffield Department of Population Health, University of Oxford,
Old Road Campus, Headington, Oxford OX3 7LF, UK
e-mail: adam.briggs@dph.ox.ac.uk; peter.scarborough@dph.ox.ac.uk;
adrian.smith@dph.ox.ac.uk

© Springer International Publishing Switzerland 2016
K. Regmi, I. Gee (eds.), *Public Health Intelligence*,
DOI 10.1007/978-3-319-28326-5_4

long to complete. Models can therefore be used to simplify reality and help public health decision makers in their day-to-day work. This chapter discusses when modelling is used, the main methodologies, and how you can criticise models through understanding their principal limitations. Chapter "Public Health Surveillance" covers public health surveillance and this will not be covered in this chapter.

Why Model?

Public health focuses on understanding the health of populations and the health effect of interventions aimed at populations. Understanding disease trends or intervention effects in populations is often more complex than for individuals. This is particularly the case where a person's health is determined by interaction with other people in the population such as in many communicable diseases. Further, public health interventions often aim to reap health benefits over very long timescales, for example, policies aimed at reducing obesity. Classical controlled experimental research designs can be unfeasible, unethical, or inadequate for such questions. Modelling has become an increasingly popular and acceptable method to circumvent the limitations of empirical methods by using existing data relevant to a public health issue to derive qualitative or quantitative insights into a distant or complex public health outcome.

For example, a commonly discussed and implemented public health policy is a tax on sugar-sweetened drinks. Randomised trials have shown that consumption of sugar-sweetened drinks causes increased body weight, and there is good experimental evidence that people's food purchasing behaviour is sensitive to changes in price. However, it is implausible to study the effect of a sugary drink tax in a randomised controlled trial. It is impractical to randomise individuals to an increase in price of sugar drinks, as they are ubiquitously available. Randomising areas to increases in price is also impractical as all vendors within the area would need to comply with the increase in price, which would require government intervention to support. Therefore, estimates of the impact of taxes on sugar-sweetened drinks are generally based on public health models.

Common areas in public health that use modelling include:

- Health service resource planning including projecting future disease burdens and resource use
- Infectious disease surveillance and control
- The potential impacts of public policy
- Cost-effectiveness of interventions or policies
- Identifying determinants of changes to disease patterns
- Testing of hypothetical 'what if' scenarios

Discussion Task
Think of a scenario where modelling has been used in your work environment. Why was modelling used instead of other data sources, for example, routine data or empirical research? Was the modelling useful?

How to Build a Model

Models are simplified versions of reality (Fig. 1). Through using readily available data, they apply mathematical relationships between input and output variables to estimate the solution to real-world problems.

There are a wide range of different model approaches that can be used, many of which are discussed in the section, "Important Model Features" of this chapter. They vary in terms of both their complexity and what they are able to simulate. Deciding upon a modelling approach will depend on several factors, principally:

(a) The output or answer required
(b) The number of influential factors to be included
(c) The data available to estimate these factors
(d) The anticipated audience and use of model outputs

Models are constructed by identifying what output is needed, and then conceptualising the model required to get to that outcome from the problem's starting point. For example, to model the effect on obesity of introducing a bicycle hire scheme, a simple conceptual model may look something like that shown Fig. 2.

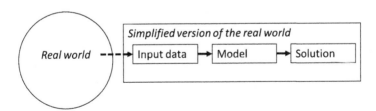

Fig. 1 How models relate to the real world. Input data and the model design are drawn from the real world (real world observed data and relationships)

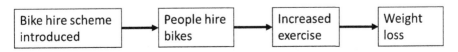

Fig. 2 A conceptual model for simulating the effect on obesity of a new bicycle hire scheme

Routinely available or specifically collected data are then needed to estimate how many people will have access to the bike hire scheme, how many are likely to hire the bikes, how much extra exercise they will do as a consequence, and how much weight loss the increased exercise is likely to lead to. Furthermore, will any of these factors vary by age and gender, or by socio-economic status and ethnicity? Routine population-level data (such as from the Office for National Statistics in the UK) can be used to identify the population who will be exposed to the scheme and their body mass index, or the modeller may choose to collect primary data to identify who is likely to access such a scheme.

Once the baseline population data are identified, models need to estimate the mathematical relationships between input variables and outcomes, and these relationships are quantified using model inputs called parameters. Generally, the mathematical relationships and the parameters make up the model structure, and this structure remains constant for all scenarios that the model is used for. For example, how much, on average, will people increase their weekly exercise if they take part in the cycle hire scheme? Such parameters are often identified from empirical research studies that have investigated such an intervention. However, in the absence of these, sometimes expert opinion is used or a certain increase in physical activity is simply assumed.

Figure 2 is clearly a very simplified example of a conceptual model. In order to more closely resemble reality, a more complex conceptual model of the same problem could look like that shown in Fig. 3, and such a model could clearly be made more complex still.

Discussion Task
1. Consider the conceptual model in Fig. 3. Do you agree with it or are the elements that you would add or remove?
2. For each parameter that the model requires (represented by an arrow), do you think that estimates are likely to be available? If not, how would you either change your model such that the step is no longer there, or how could you go about estimating the parameter?
3. Draw a conceptual model to estimate the effect on liver cirrhosis of increasing the price of alcohol. What are the major steps in the model? What data would you need both for the model's baseline data inputs and to parameterise your model?

A well-used acronym among modellers is K.I.S.S., or 'keep it simple, stupid'. In other words, models should aim to assume the simplest form that is able to adequately answer the question being asked whilst sufficiently representing the complexity of the problem. Comparing the figures above, Fig. 3 might look like a more complete representation of the possible pathways of influence between bike hire schemes and change in weight than Fig. 2. The trade-off is that increasing the number of different data inputs needed for more complicated models may mean that

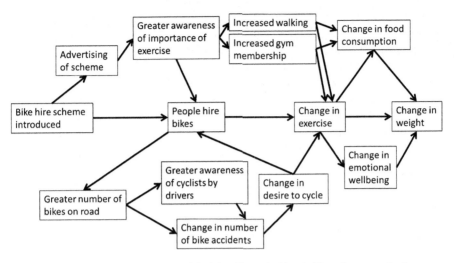

Fig. 3 A more complex conceptual model of the effect of a bicycle hire scheme on obesity

some are not backed up by robust empiric data and require guesswork (more on this can be found in section on 'Uncertainty and validity'). Finding the simplest model specification that is fit for purpose is often the most difficult and subjective task in developing models.

Important Model Features

Different modelling methods have features that make them more or less appropriate for tackling problems based on the key model influences listed at the beginning of the section on 'How to build a model'. Details of model methods are discussed in detail in the section on 'Different modelling methods', and their principle differences can be categorised by the following features.

Unit of Analysis

There are two broad ways that models simulate entire populations—as population groups or as individuals. When operating at the population level, population subgroups are often divided into one of a number of mutually exclusive health states, members of which share the same model characteristics such as rates of death or probability of moving into a different health state. For example, in relation to a sexually transmitted disease, the population at any point may be divided into population groups who are susceptible, infectious, or immune, and further subdivided into groups of different gender, sexual activity rates, or any other common feature.

By contrast, individual modelling methods simulate each individual simultaneously over time, arriving at population estimates through the aggregation of individual results. The generic term used to describe techniques that model individuals which can be aggregated to population-level outcomes is microsimulation. The model structure is the same for all individuals, but the characteristics of each individual (e.g. age, sex, blood pressure) is allowed to vary. In this way, many different characteristics can be included in the model without needing to simulate multiple population subgroups. Microsimulation also allows for individual-level interacting population structures to be applied, such as sexual networks, which may be highly relevant to disease progression in the population. However, microsimulation models generally require large amounts of input data in comparison to population models. A variety of microsimulation techniques have been used to evaluate different health policies, as discussed by Zucchelli et al., 2012.

Chance and Uncertainty

Models differ by whether or not model runs are subject to chance, and whether or not they estimate uncertainty in results. Deterministic models are those that model events without the role of chance, and which will estimate the same findings given identical parameters and starting conditions. Stochastic models refer to methods that allow modelled events to account for the effect of chance. Such models often use a random number generator to decide on the probability that is used in a particular run of the model, and overall results often summarise many model runs. Both deterministic and stochastic models can estimate uncertainty in results, and this is discussed in more detail in the section on '*Uncertainty and validity*'.

Time

Disease models often include features to mark the passage of time over which model events unfold (e.g., the estimated effect of an intervention over a period of time). Models fall into two categories by their handling of time, and model events are projected either against a continuous measure of time (often utilising differential calculus) or against discrete steps in time (such as days, weeks, or years).

Dynamic Interactions

Models can also be distinguished by whether or not the probability of a modelled event occurring is dependent on other aspects within the model which vary by time— whether there is a dynamic interaction. The ability to account for multiple population dynamics is intrinsic to many models of communicable disease, for example, the number of measles cases at a point in time may not be determined by static parameters such as transmissibility of the virus, but on dynamic parameters such as the number of susceptible and infectious individuals in the population at any point in time. By contrast, many non-communicable disease and economic processes may be appropriately modelled without dynamic components to model parameters.

Uncertainty and Validity

Models need to consider the implications to results of assumptions made in the model through estimating the uncertainty in the model's structure and its parameters, and through checking the model's validity. Important questions to ask are:

- How reliable are the data that are being used for the model's baseline values and its parameters?
- How much uncertainty is there in the model's representation of real life?

For example, suppose you were simulating the effects of food policy on cardiovascular morbidity. The model may include a parameter relating fruit and vegetable consumption to the likelihood of having a heart attack. Observational research suggests that eating three portions of fruit every day compared to just two might reduce your risk of having a heart attack in the next 10 years by 4 %. In the model, the parameter describing the proportional change in risk of heart attack for people moving from two to three portions of fruit is 0.96. Such parameters often also have an associated uncertainty, for example, when eating three portions of fruit, the risk of a heart attack in the next 10 years may potentially reduce by between 1 and 7 %. It is important to communicate this uncertainty when reporting a model's results. This is usually done by combining all the uncertainty in the model's parameters into a single 'uncertainty interval' which is presented around the central estimate of the modelled outcome.

Uncertainty

There are three main types of model uncertainty that can be analysed:

- Stochastic uncertainty
- Parametric uncertainty
- Structural uncertainty

Stochastic Uncertainty

Stochastic uncertainty analyses quantify the possibility that two individuals in identical scenarios may experience different outcomes based purely on chance alone, and can be estimated in individual-level models. For example, if two susceptible individuals spent 15 min in a room with someone infected with measles, by chance none, one, or both of the susceptible individuals may become infected. The probability of an event occurring is then drawn randomly from the true probability distribution based on a mean and standard deviation. Once a whole population has been simulated, the mean outcome can be presented alongside 2.5th and 97.5th percentiles to represent 95 % uncertainty intervals.

Parametric Uncertainty

Parametric uncertainty analyses are different in that they allow parameters in the model to vary according to the uncertainty of the parameter's estimate, based on its standard error, and can be performed in both cohort and individual models. For example, if in a model describing the spread of measles, empirical data suggest that in a susceptible population an infected person will infect 15 other people with a standard error of 1.5, the model could be rerun multiple times allowing the parameter to vary randomly according to this probability distribution. This can then be done simultaneously for all parameters in the model many thousands of times to give a probability distribution of model outcomes (often called a Monte Carlo analysis). Again, values of the 2.5th and 97.5th percentiles of the outcomes can be used to represent 95 % uncertainty intervals.

Structural Uncertainty

Quantifying uncertainty in a model's structure is more difficult—how true a representation of real life is the model? More complex models (which may be a more accurate representation of reality) require more parameters and therefore may have more parametric uncertainty (Fig. 4). Identifying the ideal model to minimise both structural and parametric uncertainty is difficult, especially since measuring structural uncertainty is challenging. This can be done through developing multiple model structures and comparing outcomes, or through other more statistically sophisticated approaches. In practice, it often becomes an iterative approach as a model develops over time and is something that it is important to be aware of.

Sensitivity Analyses

Sensitivity analyses can be used to deterministically estimate the effect of model assumptions on the model's outcomes. These assumptions can relate to either model parameters or model structure. For example, to quantify uncertainty in the parameter estimating the effect of fruit consumption on heart attack risk, the model could be run for different estimates of this parameter. In this example, the model of food policy and heart attack risk could be repeatedly simulated for different values of the effect of fruit consumption on heart attack risk, for example, a 1, 3, 5, and 7 % reduction. Similarly, in the bike hire example in Fig. 3 there may be limited data to inform the modeller whether a greater awareness of the importance of exercise truly leads to increased

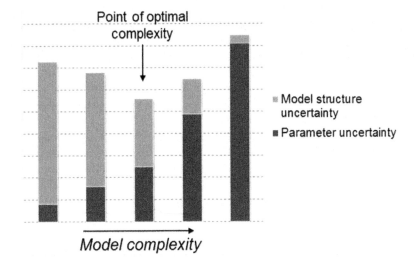

Fig. 4 Changes in parametric and structural uncertainty with increasing model complexity. Reprinted with permission from Zelm and Huijbregts, Environmental Science and Technology, 2013;47(16):9274–9280. Copyright 2013 American Chemical Society

gym membership. Sensitivity analyses could be used to estimate the effect on the model's outcome of including or not including this part of the model's structure.

In some cases, large changes in the input value (such as a specific parameter) only make small changes in the modelled output, and the model is said to be 'insensitive' to the assumed input variable. However, when large changes in the input variable lead to large changes in the modelled output then the model is said to be 'sensitive' to the assumed input variable.

> **Discussion Task**
> What are the key assumptions you have made in your conceptual model for estimating the effect on liver cirrhosis of increasing the price of alcohol (see previous Discussion Task)? How could you test these with sensitivity analyses?

Validity

Validating a model helps the model developer and model users to identify how accurately the model represents reality. The main types of validity that can be assessed are:

- Face validity
- Internal validity
- Prospective validity
- External validity

Face validity

Face validity involves sharing the model structure with people who are familiar with the system being modelled. These people are then asked whether they think that the model structure is an accurate representation of the real-life system, and to identify what steps in the model are either missing or are subject to unreasonable assumptions. Such feedback can be used to help redesign the model to improve its face validity. The model can also be run with some routine scenarios to check whether outputs are within the expected range, for example, if modelling the effects of a cancer screening programme, does increasing the number of people eligible for screening in the model lead to more diagnoses? If not, the model would lose face validity and the problem would need to be identified and corrected.

Internal Validity

Assessing a model's internal validity involves testing a model's assumptions against the data used to parameterise the model. Testing the model against the same data used to parameterise the model involves seeing if the model can replicate the observational or trial data that was used when building the model. This is a way of internally checking whether the model's structure and parameter distributions are appropriate. The model's structural validity (a type of internal validity) can also be assessed by comparing outcomes from different models testing the same problem. Models can then be analysed to identify why results may differ and how they can be improved to better represent reality. A further mechanism to internally validate the model and its parameters is to use extreme values and check that the model outputs remain reasonable. For example, a model simulating the effects of dietary fat intake on health could be run with either 0 % of calories coming from fat and then again with 100 % of calories. If such scenarios produce implausible results, then the model can be redesigned to correct the problems in the model driving such results.

Prospective Validity

Prospective validity is an extension of internal validity; this involves comparing model outputs against data from a new period of follow-up of the same datasets used to parameterise the model. Testing against these new data allows some understanding of how the model performs over time, assuming the model has a time component. As with internal validity testing, this does not offer information about any problems with the population modelled or the intervention being investigated because this is assessing validity against identical data to that used to inform the model.

External Validity

This can be thought of as the gold standard for assessing model validity and involves comparing model results with external datasets not used in the development of the model. This can only be done where such data are available, and often the reason for modelling in the first place is because empirical data do not exist. Therefore, external validation often takes place against population cohorts in different settings subjected to slightly different interventions to those simulated. This provides a key test of the model's structure and assumptions. Models that forecast changes to health over time can often be validated against historical datasets; however, it is important to understand limitations in the data against which a model is validated. For example, the quality of data collection may have changed over time or diagnostic criteria may have changed. Both may mean that the mismatch between your model's outcomes and the historical dataset is due to the historical dataset rather than a poorly performing model.

Different Modelling Methods

Modelling methods can be categorised in many ways based on the features outlined (see above). Table 1 divides some of the methods that are commonly used in public health modelling by unit of analysis (population or individual), and those that allow for dynamic interactions and those that do not.

Each of these models has different advantages and disadvantages, as discussed in more detail below (including an example of their use), and outlined in Table 2. It is important to note that many public health models will use more than one method in the same model thereby removing some the limitations of individual methodologies. Furthermore, the methods outlined below are by no means exhaustive.

Decision Tree Analyses

Decision tree analyses are often used in health economic modelling to estimate how both morbidity and costs would change following an intervention. In health technology appraisals, such as those published by the National Institute for Health and Care

Table 1 Different public health model structures (adapted from Brennan et al., 2006)

	Population level	Individual level
No dynamic interaction allowed	Decision tree analyses	Decision tree analyses
	Comparative risk assessment	Markov models
	Markov models	Multistate life tables
	Multistate life tables	
Dynamic interaction allowed	Markov models	Markov models
	System dynamic models	Discrete event simulation
		Agent-based simulation

Table 2 Advantages and disadvantages of different modelling methods

Modelling method	Advantages	Disadvantages	Example
Decision tree	Can be easy to construct	No explicit time component	Comparing exercise referral schemes with usual care to increase physical activity (Trueman and Anokye, 2013)
	Relatively easy to interpret	Exponentially more complex with additional disease states	
	Can be adapted for populations and individuals	No looping/recurring	
	Can simulate parametric uncertainty	Poorly suited to complex scenarios	
Comparative risk assessment	Can model multiple diseases and risk factors simultaneously	More complex to build than decision trees	The Global Burden of Disease Project estimating the attributable risk of risk factors for different disease outcomes (GBD 2013 Risk Factor Collaborators, 2015)
	Can estimate parametric uncertainty	No explicit time component	
	Can be used for individuals or populations	No looping/recurring	
		Unable to model dynamic interactions	
Markov models without interaction	Relatively straightforward to construct and to communicate	The Markovian assumption—individuals have no memory of (are independent of) previous disease states	Investigating the cost-effectiveness of different smoking cessation strategies using the Benefits of Smoking Cessation on Outcomes (BENESCO) model (Howard et al., 2008), and the US Centre for Disease Control model evaluating the cost-effectiveness of different diabetes prevention strategies (Herman et al., 2005)
	Can model populations or individuals	Can only exist in one disease state	
	Can simulate parametric uncertainty	Exponential increase in complexity with increasing numbers of disease states	
	Has time component		
	Allows looping/recurring		
	Can allow for dynamic interactions		
Multistate life tables	Can be used with comparative risk assessment and decision tree models to add a time component	Assumes diseases are independent of each other	The Australian Assessing Cost Effectiveness (ACE) project (Cobiac et al., 2009)
	Can be combined with Markov models to increase the numbers of possible disease states without exponentially increasing model complexity	Model limited by underlying model structure, for example, if combined with a Markov model, the Markovian assumption remains	

Model type	Advantages	Disadvantages	Examples
System dynamics models	Allows for interactions between populations and the environment Allows for feedback and recurring	Dynamic component of model is deterministic and its variability cannot be stochastically modelled Models populations rather than individuals	Generating hypotheses about the potential impact of funding changes and GP assessment rates on the health and social care system (Wolstenholme, 1993)
Ordinary differential equations models	Allows for interaction between populations and the environment Allows for feedback Uses differential equations to estimate unknown model variables	Models populations rather than individuals Difficult to estimate multiple outcomes and multiple unknown variables	Estimating the reproduction number of Ebola virus (Althaus, 2014)
Discrete event simulation	Allows for interaction between individuals and between individuals, populations, and their environment, governed by system rules Can model parametric uncertainty Allows for modelling of complex scenarios	Model structure can be difficult to communicate and interpret Computationally challenging both in terms of designing the model and running it	Evaluating the cost-effectiveness of screening programmes (Stout et al., 2006)
Agent-based simulation	Allow for interactions within and between individuals, populations, and the environment, governed by rules applied to individuals Allows for individuals to learn Allows modelling of complicated systems	More complex than discrete event simulation Requires large computational power	Understanding the possible effects of social networks on communicable disease outbreaks (Eubank et al., 2004)

Excellence (NICE), these often evaluate new drugs. However, decision tree analyses can also be used to investigate public health interventions such as the costs and consequences of introducing exercise referral schemes (Trueman and Anokye, 2013).

Branches are used to diagrammatically represent events with each branch point (or node) representing either a decision or a chance event. Each chance event has a probability of occurring such that all branches immediately following a chance node add up to one (some event must occur), with the most distal branches from the initial decision node representing the eventual outcome (often represented as a triangular terminal node). The probability of that outcome occurring is the multiple of all the probabilities at each branch point preceding that final event. The outcome can then be assigned a morbidity score (often called a disability weight, allowing different diseases to be directly compared) and a cost of that particular set of events occurring. The cost-effectiveness of an intervention can then be calculated in a relatively straightforward manner by multiplying the costs and disabilities for each outcome with the associated probability of that outcome occurring, before adding all outcomes up for each decision (see Fig. 5 for a hypothetical example of providing bariatric surgery or dietician referral to prevent obesity-related coronary heart disease).

Decision trees can be simple both to construct and to interpret. With the appropriate software, they also allow the user to estimate probabilistic uncertainty. However, they do not allow for dynamic interactions and can become rapidly more complicated when modelling increasing numbers of coexisting disease outcomes. They also have two major limitations which can make it particularly challenging to model long-term disease outcomes and communicable diseases. Firstly, the model has no explicit time component making it unsuitable for modelling changes to diseases and disease progression over time. Secondly, decision trees do not allow for looping or recurring—this means that once an individual or population in the model has a disease, they cannot loop back to their previous non-diseased state.

Discussion Task
Draw a decision tree to show possible disease outcomes from introducing a new drug rehabilitation service in your local area.

Comparative Risk Assessment

Comparative risk assessment models are most commonly used to compare disease outcomes between populations when a risk factor is changed. A particularly well-known comparative risk assessment model is that used by the Global Burden of Disease Project to estimate the attributable risk of different behavioural, metabolic, and physiological risk factors for different disease outcomes (GBD 2013 Risk Factor Collaborators, 2015).

Comparative risk assessment models use baseline data for a population's disease burden and the prevalence of a given risk factor, for example, the average amount of fibre consumed and the burden of colorectal cancer. The parameter describing the

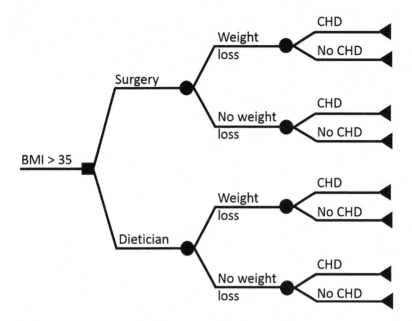

Fig. 5 A hypothetical example of a decision tree for a trial of bariatric surgery or dietician referral for individuals with a body mass index (BMI) greater than 35 kg/m². The *square* represents a decision node, the *circles* represent change nodes, and the *triangles* are terminal nodes. *BMI* Body Mass Index, *CHD* Coronary Heart Disease

independent effect of fibre consumption on colorectal cancer, often derived from observational or trial based data, can be used in the model to describe how the burden of colorectal cancer in the population would change if fibre consumption increased.

Under certain simplifying assumptions, this can be done for multiple diseases and multiple risk factors simultaneously without significantly adding to the complexity of the model. One assumption is that the parameters describing the relationships between risk factors and disease outcomes are independent of each other—the reduction in risk of getting colon cancer from increasing fibre intake is independent of the increased risk in colon cancer of simultaneously increasing consumption of processed meat. As with decision trees, comparative risk assessment models can estimate parametric uncertainty but do not allow for interaction or feedback loops, nor do they have an explicit time component (unless used in conjunction with another modelling method, such as a life tables model).

Markov Models

Markov models are used in many areas of public health modelling, and particularly in health economic modelling. In a Markov model, individuals or population groups exist in one of a limited number of disease states. At a given time point (say one year), the population being modelled moves between disease states based on pre-defined

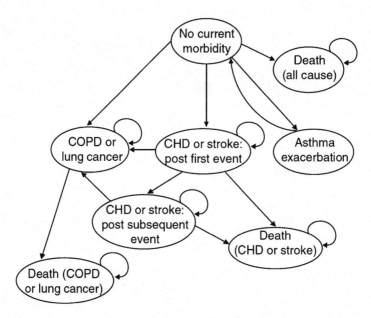

Fig. 6 Benefits of Smoking Cessation on Outcomes (BENESCO) model representation. Each *oval box* represents a diseases state, and each arrow represents a transition probability. Reprinted with kind permission from Springer Science+Business Media: Pharmacoeconomics. Cost-utility analysis of varenicline versus existing smoking cessation strategies using the BENESCO Simulation model: application to a population of US adult smokers. Volume 26, 2008, page 499. Howard, P., Knight, C., Boler, A., & Baker, C. Figure 1. Copyright 2008 AdIs Data Information BV

transition probabilities. Figure 6 is a representation of a Markov model used to estimate the effects of smoking cessation—the Benefits of Smoking Cessation on Outcomes (BENESCO) model (Howard et al. 2008). Each oval box is a disease state and each arrow represents a transition probability. Therefore at each time point, the population being modelled moves between disease states, based on the transition probability, either for a certain number of years, or until the entire population reaches a terminal state (the three death states). The arrows that arise from a disease state and loop back onto themselves represent the probability that someone stays in the same disease state, and the arrows to and from the state of asthma exacerbation is an example of recurrence or looping.

When investigating the potential effects of an intervention, such as one that means fewer people smoke in a population, the transition probabilities can either change (e.g., a smaller proportion of the population develop a smoking-related disease each year), or the population being modelled can change (e.g., if only modelling smokers, fewer individuals are modelled). If calculating the cost-effectiveness of that intervention, each disease state is assigned an associated cost and disability weight. By summing the costs and disabilities multiplied by the total number of person-years of each disease state with and without the intervention, the cost-effectiveness of the studied intervention can be calculated.

> **Discussion Task**
> Draw a diagram of a Markov model to simulate the effects of increasing the proportion of the population prescribed HMG-CoA reductase inhibitors (statin drugs) to prevent heart attacks and stroke. Also include possible drug side effects in your model.

Although the example in Fig. 6 is a relatively simple Markov model, they can be designed to incorporate large numbers of disease processes. Having said this, when adding multiple diseases that can coexist, the model can rapidly become very complicated with an exponential increase in disease states with increasing numbers of simulated diseases. Also, Markov models can be made more realistic by adding tunnel states. These are disease states that, if entered, the population or individual has a 100 % probability of exiting in the next cycle. For example, in the first year after a heart attack, the associated costs and disability are higher than subsequent years, and therefore a tunnel state called 'first year post heart attack' can be used to reflect this.

To model heterogeneous populations, i.e. populations that may have different transition probabilities, costs, and disabilities based on age, gender, or socio-economic status, two main approaches can be used. Firstly, transition probabilities, costs, and disabilities can be weighted by the proportion of the different population groups in the population being modelled. Secondly, each population group can be modelled separately with their age, gender, and socio-economic group specific transition probabilities, which allows for results to be analysed by population subgroup, as well as at the whole population level.

Further detail can be added to Markov models to allow for dynamic interactions. To do this, transition probabilities can include functions that vary with population characteristics or time elapsed. A US Centre for Disease Control (CDC) diabetes prevention Markov model developed by Hoerger et al. (see online appendix of Herman et al., 2005 for an explanation of the methods) does this by including transition probabilities that vary based on time elapsed since diabetes diagnosis, and on levels of glycaemia and hypertension—both characteristics that evolve through the model rather than being pre-defined. This model is also an example of one that deals with population heterogeneity by simulating 560 separate cohorts, with transition probabilities varying by age, sex, race, hypertension, cholesterol, and smoking status.

The fact that Markov models can be graphically communicated makes it easier for decision makers to understand the model's steps and limitations. They also allow for estimates of parametric uncertainty. However, Markov models have several important limitations, the principal one being the Markovian assumption which means the model has no memory—everyone in a disease state has the same characteristics (such as subsequent transition probabilities) irrespective of how they arrived in the state or how long they've been there. Furthermore, as with the

US CDC diabetes prevention model, models can rapidly become complex when modelling heterogeneous populations and multiple diseases whilst allowing for interaction. Models are therefore often much more simplified versions of reality (such as the BENESCO model) that may lack face validity. In order to simulate more complicated scenarios, other model structures discussed below may be more appropriate.

Multistate Life Tables

Life tables describe the probability of death from a disease for a population at different ages. For this chapter, multistate life tables are defined as disease specific tables that describe not only the probability of death from a disease, but also the age-specific probabilities of developing the disease.

These tables can be used to add a time component to decision tree and comparative risk assessment models. The age-specific probabilities of disease or death from the multistate life table can be used to parameterise repeat runs of a decision tree or comparative risk assessment model, thereby simulating a population cohort as it ages. Multistate life tables can also be combined with Markov models to overcome the need for a very complicated Markov model when simulating multiple diseases. For example, the Australian Assessing Cost Effectiveness project estimates the cost-effectiveness of different approaches to increasing population physical activity (Cobiac et al., 2009). They modelled five disease processes where the population being simulated could simultaneously exist in each disease state, which was a basic Markov model parameterised by a disease-specific life table. An overall life table then collated the results from all five diseases, summing the different disabilities and associated costs of the population being modelled. A major assumption associated with this approach, however, is that diseases are independent, i.e. the likelihood of having a stroke is independent of the likelihood of developing diabetes.

System Dynamic Models

System dynamic models are population-based models that are designed to allow for interactions between populations being modelled and between populations and the environment. Feedback loops within the model allow the system to change as the model runs, governed by algebraic or differential equations. This can be used to simulate a range of scenarios and generate hypotheses about how changing one variable may affect the wider system, for example, in health care systems. An important outcome of system dynamic models is their diagrammatic representation. This makes it easy to visualise the effect of individual variables and their related feedback loops, thereby allowing users to identify possible problematic points within the system.

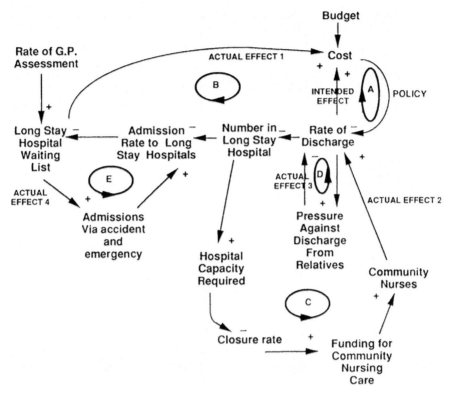

Fig. 7 Representation of the system dynamics of the UK health and social care system in the 1990s, and how the system may be affected by changes to government policy, budget, or GP assessment rates. Arrows with + symbols indicate positive association, and arrows with − symbols indicate negative association. Reprinted by permission from Macmillan Publishers Ltd: Journal of the Operational Research Society. Wolstenholme, 1993;44(9):925–934. Copyright 1993 published by Palgrave Macmillan

Figure 7 is a diagram representing the potential system dynamics of a health and social care system, taken from Wolstenholme, 1993. An arrow with a + symbol represents a positive association whereas an arrow with a − symbol represents a negative association. Loops A to E highlight possible positive or negative feedback loops within the system being modelling, and these loops will dictate how changes to government policy, the budget, or GP (general practitioner) assessment rates will affect the overall system.

Ordinary Differential Equations Models

Differential equations can be used to estimate how a variable changes with time (the variable's dynamics) and are often used as part of many dynamic models described in this chapter. Ordinary differential equations (ODE) models are used

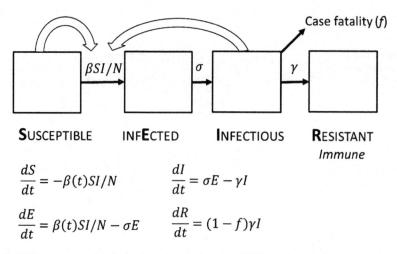

$$\frac{dS}{dt} = -\beta(t)SI/N \qquad \frac{dI}{dt} = \sigma E - \gamma I$$

$$\frac{dE}{dt} = \beta(t)SI/N - \sigma E \qquad \frac{dR}{dt} = (1-f)\gamma I$$

Fig. 8 A diagrammatic and algebraic representation of an ODE model estimating the transmission of Ebola

here to describe models that estimate how a system changes over time and are dependent on solving differential equations to derive one or more of the model's variables. Compared to system dynamic models which are often used to generate hypotheses from scarce data, ODE models may use a large amount of observed data in order to estimate the model's dynamic components through applying differential equations. They are often used in infectious disease modelling where the development of immunity and the change in the size of the remaining susceptible population affects infection rates.

Figure 8 is a diagrammatic and algebraic representation of an ODE model estimating the transmission of Ebola, as used by Althaus, 2014. Boxes represent mutually exclusive compartments representing all relevant states in the population, and the dark arrows represent the transition rates between these states or of leaving the population due to mortality. Whilst three transitions are dictated by fixed parameters (σ, f, γ), the rate of infection is influenced (white arrows) by a fixed transmission upon contact parameter (β) applied to a dynamic parameter representing the number of contacts within population. Infection rates are therefore dependent upon changes in the number of susceptible and infectious individuals over time. The rate of change of populations in each state is resolved by four differential equations, integration of which yields the number of population in each state for any value of t.

Discrete Event Simulation

Discrete event simulation is a flexible individual modelling method that simulates how a system changes over time following sequential discrete events. The system is defined by rules that dictate the probability of an event occurring, and then how the system changes on the basis of that event. Therefore, as individuals move through the model in a stochastic manner, each event that occurs can affect the probability of simultaneous events occurring and of future events. These probabilities can then vary based on an intervention being modelled.

Such models are used in a range of public health arenas, including screening, infectious disease, and health systems. Using screening as an example, Stout et al., 2006, simulated the potential population implications on diagnoses and costs of 64 different breast cancer screening protocols in the USA (varying by age invited and frequency of invites). A discrete event simulation model allowed the authors to model four major processes: the natural history of breast cancer as it develops, detection of breast cancer via screening mammography or clinical signs, improvements in treatment and treatment diffusion, and incidence of death from breast cancer or other causes. As individuals progressed through the model, based on interactions between these four processes, the authors could estimate the subsequent population-level harms and benefits of each protocol.

Although very flexible, discrete event simulation can be very complex requiring significant computational power. Furthermore, they can be difficult to represent diagrammatically and therefore to communicate to decision makers.

Agent-Based Simulation

Agent-based models are microsimulation models that allow for interactions of a heterogeneous group of individuals (agents) between each other and with the environment. They differ from discrete event simulation in that rules are applied to the agents rather than to the system. This allows for modelling of complicated systems and enables agents to learn or change over time. This feature is particularly useful when modelling social networks or infectious diseases.

An example is Eubank et al., 2004 who used agent-based simulation to analyse the effects of social networks in an urban environment on the spread of communicable disease outbreaks. The results of which can be used to simulate the impact of different outbreak mitigation strategies. However, agent-based simulation suffers from the same challenges as discrete event simulation in that large amounts of computational power are required. Also, the models can require complex social networks to be defined and parameterised, often when there are little empirical data available.

Case Study: Minimum Unit Pricing (MUP) in Scotland
Scotland was the first country in the world to introduce an MUP act for alcohol. The act sets a legally enforced minimum price at which a unit of alcohol can be sold from any premise in Scotland, with the aim of reducing harmful drinking levels.

Since Scottish devolution in 1999, leading political parties have unanimously agreed that harmful drinking in Scotland is an important public health problem, and various strategies have been developed to help tackle this.

Following the publication of a key paper in the Lancet in 2006 on the harms of alcohol in the Scottish population (Leon and McCambridge, 2006), there was an increased emphasis on tackling harmful alcohol consumption, with both NHS Health Scotland and the Scottish Health Action on Alcohol Problems (SHAAP) both highlighting the importance of price as a key determinant of alcohol misuse.

Around the same time, Sheffield University were asked by the UK Government to review the evidence and estimate the effects of different alcohol pricing interventions (including MUP) on health (Brennan et al., 2008). Such price changes would have been impossible to empirically evaluate due to the difficulty of conducting a randomised controlled trial of price changes across large numbers of retail outlets, the ethics, and challenges of recruiting potential harmful drinkers as participants, and the long time lag between the intervention and health outcome. As such, the Sheffield model was the ideal solution. Using a combination of Markov and life-table methods, the model indicated that MUP would have the greatest effect on those most at risk of alcohol-related harm, compared to general taxation approaches.

The Scottish Government asked the Sheffield team to produce a Scotland-specific analysis (Purshouse et al., 2009) and after several legal challenges, the Alcohol (Minimum Pricing) Act (Scotland) was enacted in 2012 with a minimum price of 50p per unit. Legal challenges (particularly by the Scotch Whisky Association) have meant that at the time of writing, the act is still yet to be implemented.

Conclusion

This chapter began by outlining situations where public health modelling can be useful. Important steps in building and interpreting a model were then discussed, including highlighting how models can deal with assumptions and uncertainty. Finally, some of the main modelling methods were outlined along with examples. Further information on each of the modelling methods described in this chapter can be obtained from the references. This should give you the capacity to use models more appropriately in your day-to-day work and to have the confidence to explain models to colleagues as well as understand their limitations.

Further Discussion

Modelling in public health is continuously evolving as new techniques are used and better data become available. As discussed in this chapter, public health professionals are predominantly using model outputs rather than developing their own models from scratch. For other types of research, such as trials or cohort studies, checklists or tools exist to help readers appraise the quality of the evidence (e.g., those available from the Critical Appraisal Skills Programme, or CASP: www.casp-uk.net). At the time of writing, checklists for modelling studies aren't available. Work is underway to develop reporting guidelines for non-communicable disease modelling studies, and these may provide a useful framework from which a checklist could be developed, thereby distilling much of what is found in this chapter into an easily used appraisal tool.

References

Althaus, C. L. (2014). Estimating the reproduction number of Ebola virus (EBOV) during the 2014 outbreak in West Africa. *PLoS Currents, 1.* doi:10.1371/currents.outbreaks.91afb5e0f279e7f2 9e7056095255b288.

Brennan, A., Chick, S. E., & Davies, R. (2006). A taxonomy of model structures for economic evaluation of health technologies. *Health Economics, 15*, 1295–1310.

Brennan, A., Purshouse, R., Taylor, K., Rafia, R., Meier, P. et al. (2008). *Independent review of the effects of alcohol pricing and promotion: Part B. Results from the Sheffield Alcohol Policy Model.* Sheffield: University of Sheffield. Retrieved September 23, 2015, from https://www.shef.ac.uk/polopoly_fs/1.95621!/file/PartB.pdf.

Cobiac, L. J., Vos, T., & Barendregt, J. J. (2009). Cost-effectiveness of interventions to promote physical activity: A modelling study. *PLoS Medicine, 6*, e1000110.

Eubank, S., Guclu, H., Kumar, A., Marathe, M. V., Srinivasan, A., Toroczkai, Z., et al. (2004). Modelling disease outbreaks in realistic urban social networks. *Nature, 429*, 180–184.

GBD 2013 Risk Factor Collaborators. (2015). Global, regional and national comparative risk assessment of 76 behavioural, environmental, occupational and metabolic risks or clusters of risks in 188 countries 1990-2013: A systematic analysis for the GBD 2013. *Lancet.* doi:10.1016/S0140-6736(15)00128-2.

Herman, W. H., Hoerger, T. J., Brandle, M., Hicks, K., Sorensen, S., Zhang, P., et al. (2005). The cost-effectiveness of lifestyle modification or metformin in preventing type 2 diabetes in adults with impaired glucose tolerance. *Annals of Internal Medicine, 142*, 323–332.

Howard, P., Knight, C., Boler, A., & Baker, C. (2008). Cost-utility analysis of varenicline versus existing smoking cessation strategies using the BENESCO simulation model: Application to a population of US adult smokers. *PharmacoEconomics, 26*, 497–511.

Leon, D. A., & McCambridge, J. (2006). Liver cirrhosis mortality rates in Britain from 1950 to 2002: An analysis of routine data. *Lancet, 367*, 52–56.

Purshouse, R., Meng, Y., Rafia, R., & Brennan, A. (2009). Model-based appraisal of alcohol minimum pricing and off-licensed trade discount bands in Scotland. A Scottish adaptation of the Sheffield Alcohol Policy Model version 2. Sheffield: University of Sheffield. Retrieved September 23, 2015, from https://www.shef.ac.uk/polopoly_fs/1.95608!/file/scottishadaptation.pdf.

Stout, N. K., Rosenberg, M. A., Trentham-Dietz, A., Smith, M. A., Robinson, M. A., & Fryback, D. G. (2006). Retrospective cost-effectiveness analysis of screening mammography. *Journal of the National Cancer Institute, 98*, 774–782.

Trueman, P., & Anokye, N. K. (2013). Applying economic evaluation to public health interventions: The case of interventions to promote physical activity. *Journal of Public Health (Oxford)*, *35*, 32–39.

van Zelm, R., & Huijbregts, M. A. J. (2013). Quantifying the trade off between parameter and model structure uncertainty in life cycle impact assessment. *Environmental Science and Technology*, *47*, 9274–9280.

Wolstenholme, E. F. (1993). A case study in community care using systems thinking. *Journal of the Operational Research Society*, *44*, 925–934.

Zucchelli, E., Jones, A. M., & Rice, N. (2012). The evaluation of health policies through dynamic microsimulation models. *International Journal of Microsimulation*, *5*, 2–20.

Recommended Reading

Vynnycky, E., & White, R. (2010). *An introduction to infectious disease modelling*. Oxford, England: Oxford University Press.

Webber, L., Mytton, O., Briggs, A., Woodcock, J., Scarborough, P., McPherson, K., et al. (2014). The Brighton declaration: The value of non-communicable disease modelling in population health sciences. *European Journal of Epidemiology*, *29*, 867–870.

Public Health Surveillance

Ruth Gilbert and Susan J. Cliffe

Abstract Public health surveillance enables public health practitioners to assess and monitor changes in the population's health and make recommendations for action. The systematic, ongoing collection, analysis and dissemination of data ensures that the right information is available at the right time to inform public health action. This chapter will introduce you to the key concepts and objectives of public health surveillance, and will help you to understand how effective surveillance systems are based on four basic steps: data collection, analysis, interpretation and response. This chapter will also help you to understand the advantages and disadvantages of the different surveillance systems which are used to collect information on public health. The chapter concludes with a look at how advances in technology, social media and the internet are shaping the future of public health surveillance.

After reading this chapter you will be able to:

- Describe the purpose and key features of public health surveillance
- Describe the basic steps which underpin public health surveillance systems
- Define different surveillance systems and critically compare their advantages and disadvantages

Introduction

What Is Public Health Surveillance?

Information from public health surveillance systems is used to assess public health status, track conditions of public health importance, define public health priorities, evaluate programmes and develop public health research (Lee et al. 2010).

R. Gilbert (✉)
Faculty of Health and Social Sciences, University of Bedfordshire,
Putteridge Bury, Luton LU2 8LE, UK
e-mail: ruth.gilbert@beds.ac.uk

S.J. Cliffe
Independant Consultant, St Albans, UK
e-mail: susan.cliffe@lshtm.ac.uk

© Springer International Publishing Switzerland 2016   91
K. Regmi, I. Gee (eds.), *Public Health Intelligence*,
DOI 10.1007/978-3-319-28326-5_5

Surveillance was originally defined by Langmuir (1963) as 'the systematic collection, consolidation, analysis and dissemination of data'. More recently, it has been defined as 'a core public health function that ensures the right information is available at the right time and in the right place to inform public health decisions and actions' (DH PHE Transition Team 2012). Surveillance systems are often thought of as information loops involving healthcare providers, public health agencies and the public. The cycle begins when cases of disease are reported by healthcare professionals to the public health agencies.

Although initially used to detect outbreaks of infectious diseases, public health surveillance is also an essential tool in tracking the occurrence of many non-communicable conditions such as injuries, birth defects, chronic conditions, mental illness and environmental and occupational exposure to health risks (Nsubuga et al. 2006; Buchler 2012; St. Louis 2012). Public health surveillance can also identify changes in the distribution of risk factors and can indicate if certain sectors of the population are at increased risk as a result of environmental, behavioural or other risk factors (Hawker et al. 2012). Consequently, surveillance data can provide an overview of a population's health status as well as the determinants of health (DH PHE Transition Team 2012). Additionally, surveillance can be used to evaluate or monitor existing control measures or determine the effectiveness of new health measures following their introduction (Nsubuga et al. 2006; Hawker et al. 2012).

Objectives of Public Health Surveillance

Public health surveillance forms an essential part of the public health toolkit. The specific objectives of a public health surveillance programme will depend on what information is needed, who needs it and how it will be used. Developing an effective surveillance programme will ensure a robust evidence base for public health action, programme planning and evaluation, and the development of research hypotheses. Surveillance data can be used to monitor key framework indicators at national and local levels, such as deaths and injuries on roads, alcohol-related admissions to hospital, excess winter deaths and people presenting with HIV at a late stage of infection. It can also provide valuable information for Directors of Public Health on the health of their local population and support clinical commissioning groups by providing measures of population health status, e.g. information on the incidence of sexually transmitted infections and vaccine preventable diseases, or GP and emergency department attendances. Additionally, epidemic intelligence supports health protection and emergency preparedness by facilitating rapid detection of outbreaks of infectious disease and can provide early warning of emerging threats (DH PHE Transition Team 2012).

Discussion Task

List key uses for public health surveillance data and give specific examples for each. Reflect on how this information could be used to support public health action?

Comments: Examples of how data from public health surveillance systems are used

- To measure the burden of known diseases and determinants of health in different populations
- To detect outbreak and epidemics
- To activate appropriate public health action in response to outbreaks
- To identify the natural history of diseases
- To identify new or emerging health concerns, or changes in infectious agents
- To monitor trends in disease rates and changes in associated risk factors
- To detect changes in health practice and behaviour
- To provide evidence to inform planning and implementation of public health programmes
- To support effective allocation of health resources
- To evaluate the effectiveness of control and prevention measures
- To support research

(from Lee et al. 2010; DH PHE Transition Team 2012)

Key Features of Public Health Surveillance Systems

Continuous, Ongoing Collection of Data

Public health surveillance involves the continuous, ongoing monitoring of the frequency and distribution of diseases and their risk factors. It encompasses the processes of systematic data collection, collation, analysis, interpretation and subsequent dissemination of information (DH PHE Transition Team 2012; Thacker et al. 2012). Data may be collected at a local, national or international level and are used to identify changes in patterns of disease or disease determinants within a given population against historical or geographical baselines (DH PHE Transition Team 2012). This enables healthcare providers and policy makers to determine exactly where control and prevention efforts need be focused and to target resources appropriately.

Efficient, Practical and Timely

A fundamental principle of public health surveillance is that surveillance systems should provide valid (true) information to decision makers in a *timely* manner, at the lowest possible cost (Nsubuga et al. 2006). In order to be effective, surveillance

Table 1 Criteria for identifying high-priority health events for surveillance (from Lee et al. 2010)

• Frequency	• Incidence
	• Prevalence
	• Mortality
• Severity	• Case-fatality rates
	• Hospitalization rate
	• Disability rate
	• Years of potential life lost
	• Quality-adjusted life-years lost
• Cost	• Direct costs
	• Indirect costs
• Preventability	
• Communicability	
• Public interest	

systems needs to be *efficient* and *practical*. When setting up a surveillance programme, it is important to consider exactly what information is required to avoid collecting data that will not be used, wasting both time and resources. A key purpose of communicable disease surveillance is to detect the occurrence of outbreaks or epidemics so immediate action can be taken to identify and control the source (e.g. outbreaks of food poisoning) or to enable health services to quickly implement emergency plans to deal with an increased number of patients (e.g. during an influenza epidemic). Therefore, it is essential that data are collected quickly and efficiently, providing *timely* information for action (Table 1). Most data are now collected electronically and automatically imported into databases, resulting in improved data quality and timeliness (Buchler 2012; Thacker et al. 2012). However, it is important to be aware that delays can occur at any point of a surveillance system, for example, physicians cannot diagnose some diseases until confirmatory laboratory testing has been completed.

Flexible and Acceptable

Surveillance systems need to be flexible in order to accommodate changes in operating conditions or information requirements without incurring significant additional costs. For example, case definitions, reporting forms or procedures may change. Acceptability is essential as it reflects the willingness of individuals and organisations to participate in a surveillance system. It is also important to regularly review the surveillance programmes and the information collected. Information or systems which are no longer of interest should be ended, and new systems developed to collect data on new, emerging threats to health.

Sensitive and Representative

It is essential that surveillance systems are both sensitive and representative. Sensitivity defines the ability of a system to detect the cases or other health events it is intended to detect. It also refers to the system's ability to detect epidemics and other changes in disease occurrence. Representativeness is the extent to which a surveillance system accurately portrays the incidence of a health event in a population. To generalise or draw conclusions about a community from surveillance data, the system must be representative.

Direct Link Between Outputs and Response

It is essential that there is a direct and immediate link between the outputs of surveillance systems and operational or policy response (Nsubuga et al. 2006). There is little point in collecting and analysing data if no action follows. The link between identifying a problem and the activation of an appropriate public health response should be governed and supported by local, national or international policy.

What's the Evidence?

Pre-defined criteria or trigger points based on long-term historical data can be used to activate specific public health action if the number of cases rises above a certain level. For example, 'baseline influenza activity' is the level of clinical influenza activity observed during the periods when influenza viruses are not circulating widely. Usually, in countries like the UK or the USA, there will be a 2–3-month period during the winter when the level of clinical influenza activity rises above the baseline threshold. As well as using data from laboratory confirmed cases of influenza, reports of patients visiting their GP with influenza-like illness (ILI) can be used to identify increasing rates of infection (Fig. 1). When influenza activity rises above the baseline rate, specific public health responses, such as the prescription of antiviral prophylaxis, will be triggered by pre-defined public health policies. As seen in this example, surveillance outputs should feed directly into an operational response in real time to minimise any delay in response (DH PHE Transition Team 2012).

Discussion Task

What are the key factors that can impact on the timeliness of surveillance programmes? What measures could you put in place to reduce their impact?

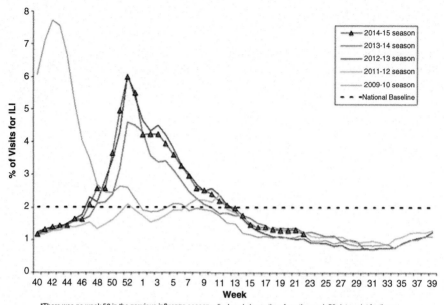

Fig. 1 A comparison of weekly reporting rates for Influenza-like illness for 2009–2015 in comparison with the expected baseline activity levels (CDC 2015)

Sources of Data

Public health surveillance data are collected from a wide variety of sources. Each source of information will provide a different overview of the frequency and distribution of disease; combining information from multiple sources can help to build up a more complete and accurate picture (Fig. 2). Most disease surveillance systems are based on anonymised reports of cases from hospital records, General Practitioners (GPs) or laboratories which are sent to a central organisation, such as Public Health England (PHE) or the Centers for Disease Control and Prevention (CDC). Valuable information is also obtained from the reporting of 'Notifiable diseases'. These are diseases that must be reported to a Government authority. Health protection legislation in the UK requires notification of approximately 30 infectious diseases. Additional surveillance data may be collected from telephone helplines, such as calls made to the NHS 111 service in England. This is called syndromic surveillance and can provide a quick indication of increased levels of symptoms, such as sickness or respiratory symptoms, in the community. Health information may also be combined with other types of data, such as demographic data collected by population surveys and environmental data.

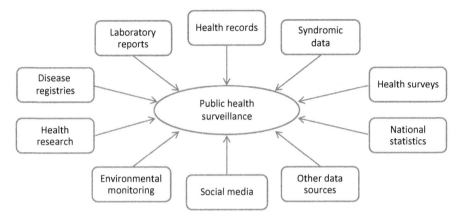

Fig. 2 Conceptual framework for public health surveillance (Adapted from Thacker et al. 2012)

Discussion Task
Suggest key sources of data which could be used in public health surveillance?

Comments: Key sources of information used in Public Health Surveillance in the UK

- Accidents and poisoning incidents
- Acute and chronic disease registers (e.g. asthma, cardiovascular disease, diabetes, mental health)
- Congenital anomaly registers
- Behaviour monitoring (e.g. smoking, diet, sexual behaviour)
- Cancer registries
- Environmental hazards monitoring
- GP episode statistics
- Healthcare-seeking behaviour, e.g. GP attendance, emergency department attendance, telehealth calls
- Horizon scanning (e.g. WHO and EWRS reports, ProMED, GPHIN, social media)
- Hospital episode statistics
- Immunisation programme data
- Infectious disease reporting
- Local authority data (e.g. Care First statistics, school, census, benefits claimants)
- Meteorological data analysis for health
- National statistics mortality data
- National Treatment Agency data (e.g. drug and alcohol use and treatment data)
- Other health determinant monitoring (e.g. obesity, poor housing, educational status)
- Screening programme data
- Termination of pregnancy statistics

(Source: DH PHE Transition Team 2012)

International Surveillance

The World Health Organization (WHO) has developed a global framework for disease surveillance, which includes formal collaborators (e.g. national public health authorities, and WHO collaborating centres and laboratories) and informal collaborators (e.g. nongovernmental organisations, including health foundations) (Thacker et al. 2012). The importance of global health surveillance increased in the late twentieth century with the emergence of HIV and novel strains of influenza (St. Louis 2012). The most important international agreement on disease control is the International Health Regulations (IHR) (World Health Organisation 2015b). Through the IHR, WHO keeps countries informed about public health risks, and works with partners to help countries build capacity to detect, report and respond to public health events. The new regulations and network were first tested when an outbreak of a novel H1N1 influenza ('swine flu') was reported in April 2009. The WHO co-ordinated the global response and the IHR effectively supported an unprecedented sharing of information between collaborating institutions and the WHO.

> **Discussion Task**
> Investigate what public health surveillance programmes currently operate in your country? Who is responsible for collecting, analysing and reporting data? Have a look at some of the key routine reports and reflect on how they are used to improve public health.

Developing Public Health Surveillance Systems

Before developing a surveillance programme a number of issues should be considered. Is the disease likely to have a negative impact on public health, for example, through causing an epidemic (e.g. influenza, cholera) or a significant public health problem (e.g. diabetes, cardiovascular disease, obesity)? Or is information required on the effectiveness of a public health intervention (e.g. immunisation programme)? It is also essential to determine whether a surveillance programme is likely to be feasible and cost-effective.

An effective surveillance system will include four basic steps: data collection, analysis, interpretation and response which will help to inform and support public health action (Fig. 3). Clear objectives and methodology need to be agreed for each programme prior to its development with the aim of optimising timeliness, representativeness and accuracy of data (Noah 2006). However, it is also essential that there is inbuilt flexibility to enable the system to adapt to changes in the population and the physical and social environment (Nsubuga et al. 2006).

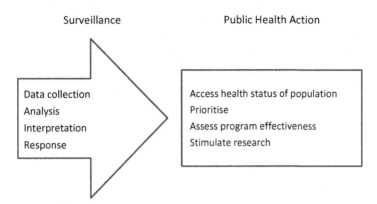

Fig. 3 A surveillance system will include four basic steps: data collection, analysis, interpretation and response (from Noah 2006)

Data Collection

Clear guidelines and case definitions are essential to ensure that all the information required is collected on a regular, timely basis. Case definitions need to be considered carefully as they will impact on the amount, type and quality of data needed. Decisions will need to be made on the optimal levels of sensitivity and specificity to balance the costs and benefits associated with false-positive and false-negative reports. Clear guidelines also help to ensure consistency and uniformity. Data can either be collected universally, covering an entire population (or a representative sample of that population) or from carefully selected locations which are deemed to be particularly susceptible to change (sentinel surveillance). The use of data standards helps to ensure that surveillance information collected over time can be compared. They can also support effective data linkage between different surveillance systems and across countries (Nsubuga et al. 2006).

Analysis

Surveillance information can analysed by time, place and person. Routine analysis is generally limited to addressing a few key important questions such as 'is the condition being reported more frequently than expected?' If so, by how much and should this trigger an 'alert'? Are cases clustered by geography or time? Does this require further investigation? It is essential to review data regularly to ensure validity (Nsubuga et al. 2006) and to ensure that the criteria for 'alert' status remain appropriate.

Simple tables and graphs are often the most useful way to summarise and present data. The use of a consistent standardised format helps to facilitate direct comparison over time. Generally, data are analysed by age and sex. However, analysis of additional variables such as occupation, sociodemographics, ethnicity and travel history may be essential in understanding the epidemiology of some diseases (Noah 2006). In some circumstances, GIS mapping can add important geographical information about the population affected or localised changes in incidence. Whenever possible, it is better to calculate disease rates than simply presenting the number of cases. However, with routine surveillance this is not always possible as the denominator (information on the size of the population) is not always available.

Interpretation

Interpretation involves converting the statistics into practical, useful information. To do this, it is essential to have a good understanding of what the surveillance system can and cannot realistically deliver. It is also important to consider timeliness of reporting and representativeness (Noah 2006). Surveillance data generally only represent the tip of the iceberg (Fig. 4). However, the proportion of cases reported is likely to depend on factors such as the severity and duration of disease. For example, most cases of meningococcal meningitis will require treatment and are likely to be reported, while only a small proportion of patients with a foodborne illness will seek healthcare (Somerville et al. 2012). However, trends in the proportion of cases that are reported for different conditions generally remain relatively constant over time. When interpreting changes in rates over time, it is important to consider whether any factors have changed within the system, for example, changes in diagnostic testing protocols or an increase in media publicity, etc. which may distort the results.

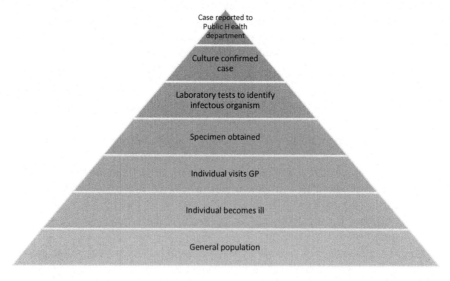

Fig. 4 The prevalence of illness pyramid (Adapted from FoodNet 1997, p. 581)

Examples of Surveillance Data Outputs

Tuberculosis Surveillance

Figure 5a presents the number of cases of tuberculosis (TB) reported in the UK by year. This simple data analysis shows whether the number of cases have changed over time. The calculation of rates takes into account denominators (or the comparative size of different populations) and therefore is useful when comparing the

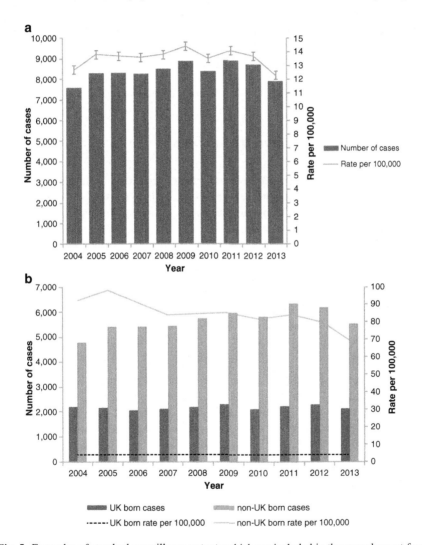

Fig. 5 Examples of standard surveillance outputs which are included in the annual report from the UK Enhanced tuberculosis surveillance programme. (**a**) Tuberculosis case reports and rates, UK, 2004–2013 and (**b**) tuberculosis case reports and rates by place of birth, UK, 2004–2013 (PHE 2014a)

number of cases in different sized groups or populations. However, this type of graph provides very little useful data for policy makers or public health practitioners since it gives no indication of whether these rates vary in different areas of the country or in different groups of the population. To address these issues, the tuberculosis surveillance programme in the UK is an 'enhanced surveillance programme' which collects information on variables such as country of birth and ethnicity, in addition to routine demographic information such as age and sex. This information can be used to help develop policies focusing on improving the health of vulnerable groups. For example, Fig. 5b shows the rates of tuberculosis in two groups of the population: those born in the UK and those born elsewhere (non-UK born). It clearly shows that the rates of infection are over 20 times higher in the non-UK born population than in UK born. If we had simply presented the number of cases the size of this disparity would not have been seen as the size of the non-UK born population is much smaller.

Reflect on how this information can be used to improve public health?

Monitoring Immunisation Programmes

Disease surveillance can be used to monitor the effectiveness of immunisation programmes. Most vaccine preventable diseases are notifiable diseases meaning that it is a legal requirement to report any cases to a Government authority (PHE in England). Figure 6 compares data from two immunisation programmes: diphtheria and measles.

Figure 6a shows that in the UK in 1914, there were approximately 60,000 diphtheria cases which resulted in approximately 6000 deaths, and that between 1914 and 1944, thousands of cases of diphtheria were reported each year. Mass vaccination was introduced in 1942 and by the early 1950s very few cases were reported. The surveillance data clearly shows that the immunisation programme in England and Wales was a success. Compare this with the data from the measles immunisation programme.

- Was the measles programme as effective initially? Reflect on why you think this may have been?
- What intervention(s) successfully reduced the number of cases of measles?
- From this graph, describe how the vaccine coverage rates have changed over time. Based on these surveillance outputs, what public health action would you propose to improve public health?

Response

Timely dissemination of data is critical to avoid a delay between the analysis of data and activation of an appropriate public health response (Nsubuga et al. 2006). The automation of reporting procedures can optimise efficiency. Since surveillance

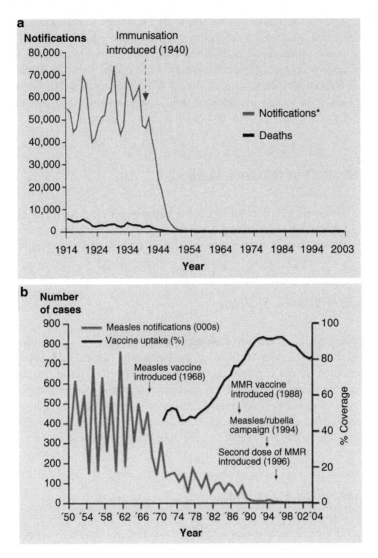

Fig. 6 Examples of surveillance data monitoring the effectiveness of immunisations programmes. (**a**) Diphtheria cases and deaths in England and Wales: 1914–2003 and (**b**) coverage of measles vaccination and measles notifications from 1950 to 2004 (PHE 2014b)

reports are used by a wide variety of professionals such as policy makers, public health specialists as well as the media and general public, reports should include straightforward tables and figures plus an explanatory commentary. The frequency of reporting will be determined by the potential impact of the disease on public health. Monthly or quarterly reporting may be appropriate for diseases where rates are changing relatively slowly. For example, rates of healthcare associated infections are reported monthly in the UK while vaccine coverage rates are reported quarterly. In some situations, more frequent reports are needed. For example during the winter, organisations such as PHE and CDC provide weekly summaries of the number of cases of influenza and other seasonal respiratory illnesses. If the number of cases is changing rapidly, such as during an influenza epidemic or pandemic, reports may be published daily; however, this is very resource intensive. Generally in-depth reports will only be provided on an ad hoc or annual basis.

Public Health Surveillance Methods

Public health surveillance data are collected in many ways, depending on the nature of the health event under surveillance, potential methods for identifying the disease, the population involved, resources available and the goals of the programme.

Passive Surveillance Systems

Passive surveillance, which involves the automatic reporting of hospital or GP records, is the most common form of public health surveillance (Noah 2006). Negative results are not reported and this type of system is ideal for monitoring trends over time for relatively common diseases. Automatic electronic reporting has the advantage of reducing costs and minimising transcriptional errors; however, the information is frequently incomplete or may include misdiagnoses. Additionally, only a minimum dataset is available which may limit its usefulness.

Active Surveillance Systems

Active surveillance is used when complete reporting is required and includes the reporting of negative diagnoses. It is generally used to collect information on uncommon diseases which are likely to cause significant public health impact, such as meningococcal infections or SARS, or when cases need to be followed up with public health interventions such as immunisation, chemophylaxis, quarantine and contract tracing. It can also be used to collect data on rare diseases such as Reye syndrome or vCJD. The system has a number of advantages over passive surveillance, such as improved sensitivity and representativeness, as well as the collection of a more detailed dataset. However, it is much more expensive and time consuming, and it would be difficult to sustain large numbers of reports for long periods of time.

Enhanced Surveillance Systems

In the UK, enhanced surveillance programmes collect more detailed information than routine surveillance. They may be used to gain a clearer understanding of the true incidence of a disease prior to the introduction of a health intervention, such as an immunisation programme, or to collect additional information on key risk factors which will assist the development of effective prevention and control strategies. For example, the enhanced surveillance of TB programme collects additional information on country of birth and ethnicity.

Behavioural Surveillance Systems

Behavioural surveillance systems focus on identifying risk factors. They collect data on any attribute, characteristic or exposure that increases the likelihood of developing an infection, disease or injury.

Sentinel Surveillance Systems

Sentinel surveillance is used to monitor common diseases. Detailed or high quality information is collected from a limited network of carefully selected, geographically dispersed reporting centres, such as GP practices or hospitals. Sentinel surveillance requires more time and resources than passive surveillance, but a well-designed sentinel system can be used to identify changes in disease trends, rapidly identify outbreaks or monitor the burden of disease in a community. However, it is important to remember that sentinel surveillance will not detect rare diseases or cases if they occur outside the catchment areas of the sentinel sites (WHO 2015a).

Syndromic Surveillance Systems

Syndromic surveillance is an innovative system which is increasingly being used in many countries to monitor public health (Elliot 2014). It is a highly sensitive system which can quickly provide information on the health of the general population. It primarily measures the number of people who contact a healthcare provider to report specific symptoms such as fever, diarrhoea and vomiting, flu-like symptoms, or heat- or cold-related health issues. Anonymised information can be collected from settings such as emergency departments (A&Es), general practices, GP out-of-hours services and walk-in health centres, as well as calls to telephone health advice lines. Data can quickly indicate changes in the number of people reporting certain symptoms.

Syndromic surveillance can be used to monitor seasonal disease trends, identify outbreaks or provide information on sudden and potentially unexpected changes in disease trends during mass gatherings. It may also successfully detect novel emerging infectious diseases (Hawker et al. 2012). Sentinel surveillance can also provide ongoing and timely information about the progress of an outbreak or public health incident. For example, which areas of the country are affected? Which age groups are most at risk? Does the severity of symptoms appear to be changing? It can also indicate when the number of cases has peaked. Conversely, syndromic surveillance can also provide reassurance about an absence of incidents during a mass gathering. The main limitation of syndromic surveillance is a lack of specificity. However, the number of people reporting specific symptoms gives an indication of the size and spread of an outbreak or incident, and if necessary, symptomatic information can be compared to data collected through more traditional reporting systems.

Discussion Task

Identify an example of each type of surveillance system described above. Briefly describe the aim of the programme. Investigate why the system was chosen and reflect on its advantages and disadvantages or limitations. How could these be overcome in the future?

Comments: Examples of different surveillance systems can be found by searching the websites of organisations such as Public Health England, CDC or WHO, or by searching for peer-reviewed publications using simple searchterms such as 'sentinel surveillance'. The aim(s) of a specific system or programme will often be stated on the organisation's website, while peer-reviewed publications may discuss its advantages and disadvantages. Reflect on the advantages and disadvantages, and propose recommendations for future action to overcome the disadvantages or limitations of the system.

Case Study: Enhancing Infectious Disease Surveillance at Mass Gatherings

Mass gatherings are defined as gatherings of more than 1000 people at a specific location, for a specific purpose (WHO and HPA 2012). An influx of people from all over the world could potentially increase the risk of disease transmission and severely strain existing health services (Soomaroo and Murray 2012; McCloskey et al. 2014). During mass gatherings, it is essential to address any health issues immediately to mitigate the threat to public health. Consequently, early identification of potential threats, occurring either in the host country or globally, is crucial in providing a timely and appropriate response. To do this, effective systems and sufficient capacity must be in place to collect, analyse and interpret information, enabling health professionals and emergency responders to act quickly to protect the public's health (HPA 2013).

(continued)

(continued)

Over 14,000 athletes participated in the London 2012 Olympic and Paralympic Games, and approximately nine million tickets were sold at venues across the UK, making the London Olympics very different to previous major events. Prior to the games, concern was expressed that London's health services may be compromised. To mitigate potential risks, established surveillance and reporting systems within the UK were enhanced and new systems were introduced. A key focus was improved timeliness, with a move from weekly to daily activity reports. The new enhanced systems included:

- Two national syndromic systems which monitored emergency department activity and calls to out-of-hours GP services, enabling 24-h monitoring of the health of local residents and visitors
- An Olympic polyclinic syndromic surveillance system
- An event-based surveillance system which recorded incidents and outbreaks from across the UK
- International Epidemic Intelligence where the UK worked with international partners such as WHO and ECDC
- Enhanced microbiology services with increased capability and capacity (McCloskey et al. 2014)

During the games, improved working practices successfully resulted in enhanced surveillance and diagnostic capability while increased resilience was achieved through better reporting, data analysis and processes. In the end, it was known with some certainty that no significant events occurred! (HPA 2013). Lessons learnt from the London 2012 Games are now being used by those planning and preparing for mass gatherings in the future.

The Future of Public Health Surveillance

Public health surveillance has evolved significantly over time. As the topics of surveillance have changed, so have the methods of surveillance which have been enhanced by rapid advances in information technology. New opportunities for strengthening surveillance capacity have arisen, many of which are based on the use of internet searches and social media (Schmidt 2012). Examples of novel surveillance programmes which have used technology to gain public health information quickly, or to obtain information which would be missed by routine surveillance, include:

- Google flu trends (https://www.google.org/flutrends/) which monitors 'flu-related' Google searches. Aggregated Google search data are used to estimate influenza activity in populations around the world in near real time (Ginsberg et al. 2009).
- Flusurvey is an Internet-based influenza surveillance project (http://flusurvey. org.uk) run by the London School of Hygiene and Tropical Medicine. It aims to

capture information from the general population, many of whom will not visit a doctor and therefore will not be captured by traditional surveillance programmes. Analysis of data for 2012–2013 has shown that Flusurvey can be used to provide reliable information to policy makers in near real time (Adler et al. 2014).

- In the USA, city public health departments have been using Twitter and online reviews to identify cases of foodborne illness which would be missed by routine surveillance programmes (Kuehn 2014; Nsoesie et al. 2014).
- In the first 100 days of the 2010 Haitian cholera outbreak, cholera-related Twitter postings were found to significantly correlate with official case data and were available up to 2 weeks earlier than data collected through official reporting structures (Chunara et al. 2012).
- Mobile phone data were used to analyse population movement following the earthquake in Haiti in 2010. It was found the movement of large numbers of people could be tracked quickly and effectively. This type of information could assist organisations in delivering an effective emergency response (Bengtsson et al. 2011).
- Similarly, during the 2014–2015 outbreak of Ebola virus disease (EVD) in West Africa, CDC collated mobile phone data from the region to map population movement. They proposed that this could provide a real time early warning of new outbreaks or clusters of EVD (BBC 2014).

Discussion Task

How could social media be used in the future to enhance disease surveillance? What are the advantages, disadvantages and ethical implications of this type of approach?

Conclusion

In this chapter, we have seen that public health surveillance is the systematic, ongoing collection, analysis and dissemination of data which enables public health practitioners to assess and monitor changes in the population's health, and to make recommendations for action at a local, national or international level. We have seen that that there are a number of different surveillance strategies; however, all surveillance systems are fundamentally based on four basic steps: data collection, analysis, interpretation and response. The ever increasing use of new technology, social media and the internet continues to shape the future of public health surveillance. However, despite advances in scope and methods, the fundamental aspects of public health surveillance remain constant, with the ultimate aim of providing information for action.

References

Adler, A., Eames, K., Funk, S., & Edmunds, W. (2014). Incidence and risk factors for influenza-like-illness in the UK: Online surveillance using Flusurvey. *BMC Infectious Diseases, 14*, 232. doi:10.1186/1471-2334-14-232.

BBC. (2014). *Ebola: Can big data analytics help contain its spread?* Retrieved July 16, 2015, from http://www.bbc.co.uk/news/business-29617831.

Bengtsson, L., Lu, X., Thorson, A., Garfield, R., & von Schreeb, J. (2011). Improved response to disasters and outbreaks by tracking population movements with mobile phone network data: A post-earthquake geospatial study in Haiti. *PLoS Medicine, 8*(8), e1001083. doi:10.1371/journal.pmed.1001083.

Buchler, J. (2012). CDC's vision for public health surveillance in the 21st century. Introduction. *Morbidity and Mortality Weekly Report, 61*(3), 1–2.

CDC. (2015). *Flu view: Weekly U.S. Influenza Surveillance Report 2014-2015 influenza season week 22 ending June 6, 2015*. Retrieved July 16, 2015, from http://www.cdc.gov/flu/weekly/index.htm#OISmap.

Chunara, R., Andrews, J., & Brownstein, J. (2012). Social and news media enable estimation of epidemiological patterns early in the 2010 Haitian cholera outbreak. *American Journal of Tropical Medicine and Hygiene, 86*(1), 39–45. doi:10.4269/ajtmh.2012.11-0597.

DH PHE Transition Team. (2012). *Public health surveillance. Towards a public health surveillance strategy for England*. Retrieved July 16, 2015, from https://www.gov.uk/government/uploads/system/uploads/attachment_data/file/213339/Towards-a-Public-Health-Surveillance-Strategy.pdf.

Elliot, A. (2014). *Syndromic surveillance: Our national insurance PHE Blog Public Health Matters, 6*th *March 2014*. Retrieved July 16, 2015, from https://publichealthmatters.blog.gov.uk/.

Foodborne Diseases Active Surveillance Network Working Group. (1997). Foodborne diseases active surveillance network (FoodNet). *Emerging Infectious Diseases, 3*(4), 581–583. doi:10.3201/eid0304.970428.

Ginsberg, J., Mohebbi, M., Patel, R., Brammer, L., Smolinski, M., & Brilliant, L. (2009). Detecting influenza epidemics using search engine query data. *Nature, 457*, 1012–1014. doi:10.1038/nature07634.

Hawker, J., Begg, N., Blair, I., Reintjes, R., Weinberg, J., & Ekdahl, K. (2012). *Communicable disease control and health protection handbook* (3rd ed.). Chichester, England: Wiley-Blackwell.

Health Protection Agency. (2013). *London 2012 Olympic and Paralympic Games summary report of the Health Protection Agency's Games time activities*. London: Health Protection Agency.

Kuehn, B. (2014). Agencies use social media to track foodborne illness. *Journal of the American Medical Association, 312*(2), 117–118. doi:10.1001/jama.2014.7731.

Langmuir, A. (1963). The surveillance of communicable diseases of national importance. *New England Journal of Medicine, 24*(268), 182–192.

Lee, L., Teutsch, S., Thacker, S., & St. Louis, M. (2010). *Principles & practice of public health surveillance* (3rd ed.). Oxford, England: Oxford University Press.

McCloskey, B., Endericks, T., Catchpole, M., Zambon, M., McLauchlin, J., Shetty, N., et al. (2014). London 2012 Olympic and Paralympic Games: Public health surveillance and epidemiology. *The Lancet, 383*(9934), 2083–2089.

Noah, N. (2006). *Controlling communicable disease*. Maidenhead, England: Open University/McGraw-Hill.

Nsoesie, E., Kluberga, S., & Brownstein, J. (2014). Online reports of foodborne illness capture foods implicated in official foodborne outbreak reports. *Preventive Medicine, 67*, 264–269. doi:10.1016/j.ypmed.2014.08.003.

Nsubuga, P., White, E., Thacker, S., Anderson, M., Blount, S., Broome, C. V., et al. (2006). Public health surveillance: A tool for targeting and monitoring interventions. In D. Jamison, J. Breman,

A. Measham, et al. (Eds.), *Disease control priorities for developing countries* (pp. 997–1015). Washington, DC: World Bank.

Public Health England. (2014a). *Tuberculosis in the UK: 2014 report*. Retrieved July 16, 2015, from https://www.gov.uk/government/uploads/system/uploads/attachment_data/file/360335/TB_Annual_report__4_0_300914.pdf.

Public Health England. (2014b). *The Green Book. Information for public health professionals on immunisation*. Retrieved July 16, 2015, from https://www.gov.uk/government/collections/immunisation-against-infectious-disease-the-green-book#the-green-book.

Schmidt, C. (2012). Trending now: Using social media to predict and track disease outbreaks. *Environmental Health Perspectives, 120*(1), a30–a33. doi:10.1289/ehp.120-a30.

Somerville, M., Kumaran, K., & Anderson, R. (2012). *Public health and epidemiology at a glance*. Oxford, England: Wiley.

Soomaroo, L., & Murray, V. (2012). Disasters at mass gatherings: Lessons from history. *PLoS Currents, 4*, RRN1301. doi:10.1371/currents.RRN1301.

St. Louis, M. (2012). Global health surveillance. *Morbidity and Mortality Weekly Report, 61*(3), 15–19.

Thacker, S., Qualters, J., & Lee, L. (2012). Public health surveillance in the United States: Evolution and challenges. *Morbidity and Mortality Weekly Report, 61*(3), 3–9.

World Health Organisation. (2015a). *Sentinel surveillance*. Retrieved July 16, 2015, from http://www.who.int/immunization/monitoring_surveillance/burden/vpd/surveillance_type/sentinel/en/.

World Health Organisation. (2015b). *International Health Regulations* (IHR). Retrieved July 16, 2015, from http://www.who.int/topics/international_health_regulations/en/.

World Health Organization & Health Protection Agency. (2012). *Disaster risk management for health factsheet*. Mass gatherings. Retrieved July 16, 2015, from http://www.hpa.org.uk/webc/HPAwebFile/HPAweb_C/1317134739452.

Recommended Reading

Centers for Disease Control and Prevention. (2012). CDC's vision for public health surveillance in the 21st century. *Morbidity and Mortality Weekly Report, 61*(Suppl), 1–40.

DH PHE Transition Team. (2012). *Public health surveillance. Towards a public health surveillance strategy for England*. Retrieved July 16, 2015, from https://www.gov.uk/government/uploads/system/uploads/attachment_data/file/213339/Towards-a-Public-Health-Surveillance-Strategy.pdf

Elliot, A. (2014). *Syndromic surveillance: Our national insurance*. PHE Blog Public Health Matters, 6th March 2014. Retrieved July 16, 2015, from https://publichealthmatters.blog.gov.uk/.

Lee, L., Teutsch, S., Thacker, S., & St. Louis, M. (2010). *Principles & practice of public health surveillance* (3rd ed.). Oxford, England: Oxford University Press.

Geographic Information Systems in Health

Kristen Kurland

Abstract This chapter describes the use of Geographic Information Systems (GIS) in public health. An overview of GIS includes a brief history, military developments, computerized GIS software, and current tools. Examples of GIS applications for international, national, state, and local public health organizations will highlight how GIS is currently used. GIS advantages and disadvantages in the fields of epidemiology, medicine, and public health will provide a context for its use in the health industry. An overview of spatial statistics and space-time analysis will illustrate advanced GIS functions used by researchers and scientists for better understanding of spatial patterns, improved decision-making, and determining the statistical significance of spatial modelling.

After reading this chapter you will be able to:

- Understand the history and current uses of GIS
- Identify applications, advantages, and disadvantages of GIS for public health
- Have a basic understanding of spatial statistics for public health applications

GIS Overview

Definition

Geographic Information Systems (GIS) is a computerized system designed for the storage, retrieval, and analysis of geographically referenced data. GIS uses advanced analytical tools to explore at a scientific level the spatial relationships, patterns, and processes of biological, cultural, demographic, economic, geographic, and physical phenomena.

K. Kurland (✉)
H. John Heinz III College and School of Architecture, Carnegie Mellon University, 5000 Forbes Avenue, Pittsburgh 15213, PA, USA
e-mail: kurland@cmu.edu

© Springer International Publishing Switzerland 2016   111
K. Regmi, I. Gee (eds.), *Public Health Intelligence*,
DOI 10.1007/978-3-319-28326-5_6

Early Health Maps

While the roots of cartography go back hundreds of years, the first known GIS related to health were hand drawn maps by Dr. John Snow during a cholera outbreak in London in 1854. Snow questioned the popular theory that cholera was an air-borne miasma contagion and suspected that local cases were instead the result of a contaminated water pump on Broad Street in central London. As a physician, Dr. Snow treated many of those who died from the cholera outbreak in this area and was familiar with the neighbourhood and its citizens. Snow not only mapped the location of each death, he placed a horizontal bar for every person who died, thus demonstrating a clustering and quantity of deaths near the pump. His maps showed that no deaths occurred at a nearby pub or at an adjacent monastery where bar patrons and monks did not drink water from the Broad Street pump. However, these original maps did not convince the Board of Guardians that the pump was the cause of the cholera deaths, so Snow created a second map, an irregular line drawing showing a catchment area of those living closest to the pump. These maps showed that most of the cholera deaths were within this catchment area, finally convincing the Board of Guardians to disable the pump. The number of cholera cases declined, and water borne transmission of cholera was later established, not by Snow but by others, solidifying germ theory. John Snow is credited as a founder of the field of epidemiology and has a tavern named after him.

Around the same time but across the pond others were creating maps for studying health conditions. The New York City Metropolitan Board of Health was one of the first modern municipal public health authorities in the United States to use maps to understand the health and living conditions of the population. Figure 1 depicts health department maps of NYC's fourth ward from 1864 showing that sanitary conditions at this time were overwhelmingly poor. Yellow structures on the map show tenement houses where the space for each occupant was less than 800 cubic feet. In this year, there were 486 tenement houses with 3636 families and a total population of 17,611. There was a population of 346 living in cellars and 151 tenements without sewers (Lubove 1963). This early mapping clearly helped city officials and the Board of Health understand and ultimately improve the health and living conditions of the population.

Aerial Photography and Military Developments

GIS as used today has its roots in photography and military uses. Remote sensing, a source of GIS map creation, is the technique of collecting information about the earth from a distance. The technical development of remote sensing began with aerial pho-tography and by the 1860s photographs were taken from captive balloons. The first military use of aerial photos was June of 1862 during the American Civil War when photographs were taken by the US Army to analyse the defences of the city of Richmond. By the 1900s technology improved to a point where smaller cameras

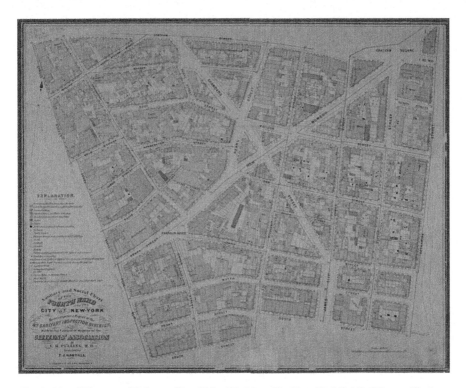

Fig. 1 Lionel Pincus and Princess Firyal Map Division, The New York Public Library. 'Sanitary and social chart of the Fourth Ward of the City of New York, to accompany a report of the 4th Sanitary Inspection District'. *Source*: The New York Public Library Digital Collections. 1864. http://digitalcollections.nypl.org/items/fc8b9560-f3a1-0130-679f-58d385a7b928)

with faster lenses were used. In 1909 Wilbur Wright was credited with taking the first photograph from an airplane and soon thereafter German flying students trained at English flying schools were taking air photos. Military authorities in WWI were initially reluctant to use aerial photography technology, but when semi-official photographic missions produced air photos of military facilities in German-held territories, they were quickly convinced of their potential use (Arnoff 1995). Figure 2 shows how mosaic maps were made by taking a series of overlapping vertical photos and aligning them together to create a comprehensive view of the enemy's trench network (Gettinger 2014). Photo interpreters became the 'eyes of the armed forces', and the use of aerial photos had a profound effect on military tactics by finding visual clues that might denote changes in the enemy's position. Examples include soil displacement or shadows to identify trenches, embankments, artillery batteries, and troop movements (Arnoff 1995).

After WWII, aerial photography technology improved due to higher flying aircraft such as the U2. These military spy planes were out of reach of most land weapons and allowed the United States to use aerial photography during the 'Cold War' (Arnoff 1995). On 24 October 1946, rocket-borne cameras launched from the White

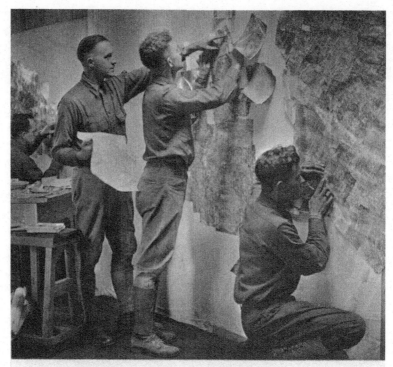

"Mosaic mapping." U.S. School of Aerial Photography, Langley Field, Virginia. (*Photo courtesy of U.S. Air Force*)

Fig. 2 'Mosaic mapping' US School of Aerial Photography, Langely Field, Virgina. *Source*: US Air Force, http://dronecenter.bard.edu/files/2014/01/00001490-1.jpg

Sands Missile Range/Applied Physics Laboratory in the New Mexico desert gave us the first look at the Earth from beyond the atmosphere (Reichhardt 2006).

Early Computerized Years

Roger Thomlinson, an English geographer, is known as the father of GIS for his involvement with the Canadian Geographic Information System, the first computerized GIS. After his military service in the Royal Air Force (1951–1954), Dr. Tomlinson received separate undergraduate degrees in geography and geology. It was during his time with the Canadian federal government in the 1960s that Tomlinson initiated, planned, and directed the development of the Canada Geographic Information System, one of the first known GIS applications for land use (Sampson 2014).

Many of today's GIS computerized technologies stem from the work done by Howard T. Fisher and his graduate students at the Harvard School of Design

Laboratory for Computer Graphics and Spatial Analysis. Most notable are Jack Dangermond, founder of Esri, Inc. (Environmental Systems Research Institute), Scott Morehouse, Hugh Keegan, and Duane Niemeyer of Esri, David Sinton of Intergraph, and Lawrie Jordon and Bruce Rado, founders of ERDAS. Applications created by these individuals encompass most of the current vector and raster technologies in use today (Hoel et al. 2009). Of these, the most dominant GIS software vendor is Esri, with 41 % of the GIS market, far more than any other GIS vendor (Esri and Jack Dangermond 2015). Its software, ArcGIS, is used by almost every US Federal agency; over 350,000 organizations globally; the 200 largest cities in the US; two-thirds of the Fortune 500 firms; and more than 7000 colleges and universities (Esri customers 2014). Esri has relationships with over 65 software, technology, data, hardware, system integrator and consulting companies including Amazon Web Services, AT&T, Citrix, IBM, Microsoft, Oracle, SAP, Nokia, and SAS (Esri partners 2013).

GIS Data

GIS data is in three formats: vector, raster, and tabular. Vector maps have features drawn using points, lines, and polygons (a polygon is a closed area that has a boundary consisting of connected straight lines) to represent discrete geographic objects such as automobile accident locations, streets, and counties. Raster maps are generally aerial photographs, satellite images, or representations of surfaces such as elevation, which are used to represent continuous geographies (Kurland and Gorr 2014). Tabular data is in the form of rows and columns such as spreadsheets and much of this data is created directly by organizations. For example, private and public health care agencies map address data from patient medical records or surveys. Common sources of tabular data are freely available from organizations such as the Australian Bureau of Statistics, the UK Office of National Statistics, the US Census Bureau and similar government organizations worldwide. These, and other local governments, are sources of business, demographic, economic, environmental, and other data used in GIS.

Data and the method for collecting and providing it have come a long way since early census taking. When it first began, the US Census sought very basic population information, but a significant change occurred in the 1940s, when the Census Bureau introduced statistical sampling. Processing and tabulation technology took a great leap forward during World War II, when the War Department began to explore the use of electronic digital computers to process ballistic information and after the war, many of the project's engineers recognized peacetime benefits of such a device. In 1943, the US National Defense Research Council (NDRC) approved the design and construction of the Electronic Numeric Integrator and Computer (ENIAC) used by the War Department's Ballistic Research Laboratory. During this project, programmers met with several Census Bureau officials to discuss non-military applications for electronic computing devices; and in 1946, programmers began work on new a computer designed for use by the Census Bureau. The final results were specifications for the Universal Automatic Computer (UNIVAC). Their efforts brought the US Census Bureau into the computer age and laid the foundation for the census data as we know it today (Univac 2015).

Before the 1960s most maps were in hard copy form. Advances in optics, metallurgy, and industry during the eighteenth and nineteenth centuries allowed the mass production of surveying devices and by the mid-twentieth century cartometric quality maps were accurately representing objects on the earth's surface. Other advances improving digital data used in GIS were Global Navigation Satellite Systems (GNSS) such as the US Global Positioning System (GPS). Optical scanning and manual digitizing (the process of collecting digital coordinates) became commonplace in the 1980s when many organizations began implementing GIS (Bolstad 2008).

Discussion Task
What tabular data could be surveyed or otherwise downloaded or created for a GIS public health study?
  Discuss

Current and Future GIS Technologies

Aerial imagery, manual digitizing, remote sensing, satellites, and scanners are technologies used to create GIS map layers. Computer software of the 1970s, 1980s, and 1990s used to develop GIS data include Computer Aided Design (CAD), vector, and raster GIS. Companies such as Autodesk, Esri, Erdas, and Intergraph, and Pitney Bowes are among those who led the way in developing software applications. Tools were added for advanced spatial analysis and many of these required specialized knowledge and advanced training.

Open source GIS applications were first developed in the 1970s and 1980s and they continue to grow. Geographic Resources Analysis Support System (commonly referred to as GRASS) is a free and open source GIS used in academic, commercial, and governmental agencies for over 30 years. GeoDa is another open source GIS commonly used for spatial regression. Spatial regression not only asks where something occurs, but why it occurs. For example, GIS shows where higher than expected traffic accidents happen in a city but regression answers what factors contribute to accidents. Spatial regression allows one to model phenomena to better understand them and predict values at other places and times (Murak 2013). QGIS, an official project of the Open Source Geospatial Foundation (OSGeo), is a more recent open source GIS. QGIS runs on Linux, Unix, Mac OSX, Windows, and Android and supports numerous vector, raster, and database formats and functionalities (QGIS 2015).

Google Maps, Google Earth, Google Earth Pro, and Microsoft Virtual Earth (formerly Bing Maps) have had a strong impact on the field of GIS. The ease of viewing satellite imagery, maps, terrain, and 3D street views has greatly increased the awareness of the geospatial industry by the general public.

Technologies such as GPS and social media as well as cloud and mobile technologies are changing the way organizations collect and analyse location-based data. The new modality of GIS is the seamless integration of desktop GIS, mobile devices, and the Web. GIS maps, workflows, and analytic data models are now shared online with many and integrated as a system. Esri's next generation of ArcGIS Platform allows users to design, edit, and publish GIS data anywhere, anytime, and from any device. Maps created in 2D and 3D from a desktop GIS can be easily published directly to Esri's ArcGIS Online or Portal. Maps can then be downloaded and viewed on mobile devices and tables. A new tool such as Esri's Collector for ArcGIS collects and updates field data on iOS and Android devices. These technologies, plus advances in medical record integration and surveys, will have a great impact on public health mapping.

GIS Applications in Public Health

Introduction

GIS has been widely used by government agencies since the 1970s and has made more recent strides into health care in both the private and public sectors. It provides an effective way to visualize, organize, and manage a wide variety of information including administrative and medical data, social services, and patient information. Public health organizations at the international, national, state/province, and local level use GIS to map health events, identify disease clusters, investigate environmental health problems, and understand the spread of communicable and infectious disease.

International Application

Organizations collecting, mapping, and spatially analysing international health data include the Kaiser Family Foundation, World Health Organization (WHO), the World Bank, and many more. The US Agency for International Development (USAID) and President's Emergency Plan for AIDS Relief (PEPFAR) are examples of agencies working together and with various countries to solve public health problems using GIS. Both are large components of the US President's Global Health Initiative. PEPFAR was established by presidential order to help educate and save the lives of those suffering from HIV/AIDS. Its goals are to strengthen the capacity of partnering governments to respond to and create sustainable programmes to prevent and treat HIV/AIDS and other infectious epidemics. USAID is responsible for administering civilian foreign aid and operates in Africa, Asia, Latin America, and Eastern Europe.

Health and family planning is a field mission of USAID, whose projects strengthen the public health system by focusing on maternal-child care health.

PEPFAR and USAID created the Spatial Data Repository to link geographic health data to demographic data provided by The Demographic Health Surveys (DHS) Program and the US Census Bureau. Since 1984, the DHS Program has worked with over 90 countries to develop more than 300 surveys to improve our understanding of the health of developing countries. Data from the surveys include fertility, family planning, maternal and child health, gender, HIV/AIDS, malaria, and nutrition. Over the past six decades the US Census Bureau has worked internationally with over 100 countries on a variety of topics used for disaster and humanitarian relief planning. Working with PEPFAR and developing country counter parts, the US Census Bureau provides population and age/sex estimates, technical help, software products, and training to assist countries in the collection, processing, analysis, dissemination, and use of statistics to better understand public health conditions (US Census 2015).

The DHS Program's Spatial Data Website (spatialdata.dhsprogram.com/home/) provides online maps as well as data that can be downloaded and used for advanced analysis using desktop GIS. Its STAT compiler application allows users to make customized tables, charts, line graphs, thematic maps, and scatter plots and has a mobile app for the 25 most popular health indicators for over 90 counties and 250 existing surveys. Figure 3 is an example downloaded DHS data mapped using Esri's ArcGIS application (Kurland and Gorr 2014). The map compares women who tested positive for HIV/AIDS and the percentage of women with no education.

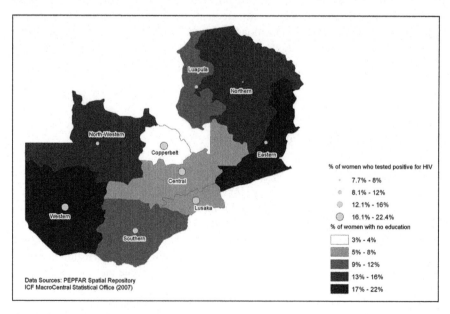

Fig. 3 Zambia HIV study of women age 15–49. *Source*: PEPFAR Spatial Repository, Kurland and Gorr (2014), GIS Tutorial for Health, Esri Press, 5th Edition, 178

National Application

National organizations collecting data for public health use vary by country. Examples are the Australian Institute of Health and Welfare (aihw.gov.au), the UK's Health and Social Care Information Centre (hscic.gov.uk), and the US Centers for Disease Control (CDC) (cdc.gov). Another US organization with strong data and GIS applications is the National Cancer Institute (NCI). For many years, NCI has provided data, maps, and advanced statistical tools via their website (gis.cancer.gov). Geospatial data from the NCI come from many sources including the National Center for Health Statistics, the Census Bureau, and lifestyle data from the CDC. Related collaborative research includes Surveillance, Epidemiology and End Results (SEER) Cancer Registries (Rapid Response Surveillance Studies). The SEER program funds special research studies by its cancer registries on topics of interest to NCI and cancer registries in general. In addition to online mapping, the NCI offers a variety of spatial statistic modelling tools, advanced geovisualization, and georeferenced statistics (National Cancer Institute 2015).

State Application

States and provinces use GIS for public health decision-making. California is the most populous state in the US, and public health officials must deliver a health care delivery system that meets the needs of its citizens. One tool designed to do this is the California Healthcare Atlas, developed and maintained by the Office of Statewide Health Planning and Development (OSHPD). In its early years OSHPD produced data that was used mostly by policy makers, researchers, or administrators with high level analytic skills. Data was stored in silos and not easily available. Today's California Healthcare Atlas provides more than 16,000 searchable, cross-referenced geographic locations related to health care in a single source Web portal. The average citizen looking for the nearest hospital, a public health official wanting to learn more about population insurance coverage, or a health policy maker needing data about health care finances or workforce, or hospitalization and discharge data can each find many of the necessary materials within the Atlas (Healthcare Atlas 2015).

Local Application

Local public health agencies use GIS for mapping and analysing health related information. One of the leaders in these efforts is the New York City Department of Health and Mental Hygiene (DOHMH), hosting an online GIS Center. Evidence of the growing connection between basic GIS mapping and advanced spatial analysis, the GIS Center uses a number of products including ESRI's ArcGIS, Google Earth,

SaTScan, FleXScan, GeoDa, and R. The GIS Center is led by a GIS Working Group (GISWG) that comprises GIS users throughout the organization and serves as a liaison for other GIS users in New York City including the NYC Office of Emergency Management, and other New York City inter-agency GIS groups. Most notably, the GIS Center collaborates with the NYC Bureau of Epi Services, Division of Epidemiology, and Division of Informatics and Information Technology (DITI) (NYC DOHMH 2015).

Important sources of data for the GIS Center are public health surveys. Each year, the Community Health Survey queries a representative sample of New Yorkers about their health. Additional surveys focus on public high school students via the Youth Risk Behavior Survey and a large group of persons who were exposed to airborne pollutants associated with the attack on the World Trade Center (2001) are followed via a health registry. A more costly survey, the NYC Health and Nutrition Examination Survey, involves a small sample of New Yorkers who participate by answering questions about nutritional patterns plus undergoing a physical exam. The Health Department also uses surveys provided by state or national organizations including the Centers for Disease Control (CDC) National Center for Health Statistics and Behavioral Risk Factor Surveillance System. Data and tables can be downloaded and used in desktop GIS applications or interactive tools can be used on the Department of Health's website to learn more about the environment, health, behaviour, and population of New York City.

Discussion Tasks

What is a possible use of GIS for a global or local public health organization?

Give an example of GIS layers used for a public health study.

Advantages and Disadvantages

Advantages

'Public health' can be defined as 'the art and science dealing with the protection and improvement of community health by organized community effort and including preventive medicine and sanitary and social science'. Today's public health organizations require multidiscipline collaborations among architecture, biology, business, computer science, education, engineering, epidemiology, medicine, public policy, sociology, and other domains. In fact, it could be argued that the most significant advances in medicine and public health over the last two centuries were due to sanitary improvements through civil engineering rather than by medical 'breakthroughs'.

GIS is an essential tool used by many of the above disciplines, enabling public officials and policy makers to better understand their citizens, environment, and

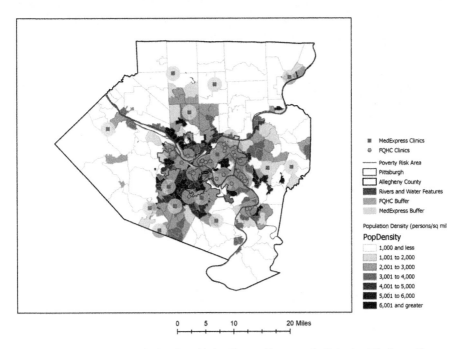

MedExpress Clinics
FQHC Clinics
Poverty Risk Area
Pittsburgh
Allegheny County
Rivers and Water Features
FQHC Buffer
MedExpress Buffer

Population Density (persons/sq mil
PopDensity
1,000 and less
1,001 to 2,000
2,001 to 3,000
3,001 to 4,000
4,001 to 5,000
5,001 to 6,000
6,001 and greater

0   5   10   20 Miles

Fig. 4 Poverty Areas, Population Density by Census Tracts, and clinics in Allegheny County Pennsylvania. *Source*: Gorr and Kurland (estimated 2016), GIS Tutorial Basic Workbook for ArcGIS Platform

communities and, with this information, to identify and solve potential problems or hazards. One example of the use of GIS is in the area of access to health care for at-risk populations. Populations living in poverty must often rely heavily on public transportation. If clinics or other medical facilities are not located in areas where at-risk populations live, or if access to adequate public transportation is lacking in these neighbourhoods, these populations have been shown to have poor health outcomes (Syed et al. 2013). By combining clinic and population data in a visual format, GIS can illustrate complex relationships affecting health care delivery; this allows for improved evaluation of policy interventions, informs health services research, and guides health care planning (Phillips et al. 2000).

Figure 4 illustrates how multiple GIS layers are used to identify health care access in low income areas in Allegheny County, Pennsylvania. US Census data shows areas of poverty and population density compared with locations of Med Express (private for profit urgent care health facilities) and Federally Qualified Health Clinics (FQHC), which under Section 330 of the Public Health Service Act must provide health services to an underserved area or population. The map shows that FQHC are located in areas affected by poverty while Med Express locations tend to be in areas of lower population density less affected by poverty. One mile GIS buffers placed around each clinic demonstrates relative access.

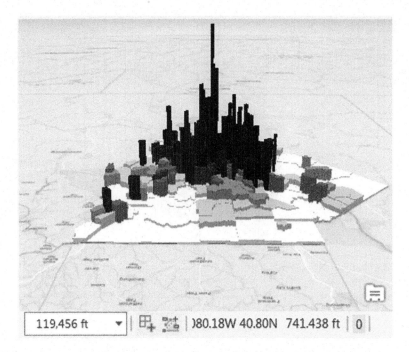

Fig. 5 Health Care Clinics 3D. *Source*: Gorr and Kurland (estimated 2016), GIS Tutorial Basic Workbook for ArcGIS Platform

Another GIS advantage is the ability to visualize data in three dimensions (3D). Population density throughout an urban area varies widely, and it is difficult to depict this merely with colour coding on a map. In 3D, the differences in density are easily appreciated, and new tools in GIS make this a seamless effort as shown in Fig. 5.

A crucial benefit of GIS for public health organizations is in its ability to inform and educate partners and communities in a way that will help them identify and solve problems. Maps can be very powerful communication tools, especially when showing the linkages between multiple variables, indicating areas of interest or concern, or when showing geographic data over time. Because maps can deliver messages without much text, they are versatile for communicating health issues; however, maps themselves are not always completely understood and written explanation is often needed, especially for the general public. Previously, maps were sometimes difficult to understand because narrative text was missing. Story Maps, combining text with maps, images, and multimedia content, are now available to better engage audiences with public health data, analysis, and projects (Esri storymaps 2015). Along with story maps, the ability to publish maps on the Web or mobile devices further enables public health organizations to share information about its communities.

GIS can serve as early warning tools. Environmental information can be used to track and potentially predict future public health needs. For example, mapping environmental factors associated with known areas affected by malaria may give insights into other areas where malaria may be occurring but is currently not well reported. Other examples include mapping forest fires as an indication of air pollution, and mapping flood-prone areas as predictors of potential cholera outbreaks (World Health Organization 2015).

Disadvantages

GIS is not without its critics. Some in epidemiology and public health argue that GIS mapping is an inconsequential tool used in the struggle to understand states of disease and health. Arguments are made that GIS maps are merely graphic and visual rather than statistical, thus offering little benefit for modern researchers. In medical science it is not enough to use the phrase 'it appears that' without statistics justifying those observations. 'GIS aficionados…see themselves as standing for the public health in the face of the jeering throng and as rushing out into the real world to save real lives while the stodgy, plodding scientists fussily demand more evidence' (Vinten-Johansen et al. 2003). In the example of John Snow's maps, it is clear that a greater understanding of the neighbourhood including the points of contagion at each household, network of streets, those using the Broad Street pump, and other environmental or locational attributes helped explain that the disease was waterborne (Koch 2005). At the same time, if a map is used solely as visual display it cannot predict the patterns of distribution nor does it infer causal relationships.

Lastly, the cost of creating, collecting, and analysing GIS data combined with privacy issues are potential important limitations. GIS requires specialized hardware and software, trained personnel, and often expensive and time-consuming means of acquiring, checking, interpreting, and inputting information. This is especially difficult in developing or poor nations. Surveys are costly to administer and privacy laws such as the US HIPPA (Health Insurance Portability and Accountability Act of 1996) prevent identifiable patient data for geographic subdivisions smaller than a state, including street address, city, county, precinct, zip code, and their equivalent geocodes difficult to be used without consent. Expert knowledge for satisfying a 'safe harbour' method of de-identification of data is often needed as well as project approval from Institutional Review Boards (Health and Human Services 2005). All of these issues may limit the utilization as well as the utility of GIS.

Spatial Statistics and Space Time Analysis

Spatial statistics is a field of study developed within mathematical sciences and has grown primarily by its application to disciplines such as agriculture, forestry, and mining engineering. The expansion of the use of spatial statistics resulted in the development of geostatistics. Over the past 20 years, there has been an explosion of interest in space and space-time problems. Advances in spatial statistics have resulted in the development of statistical methodologies, permitting the use of GIS more definitively into research-based fields including epidemiology, medicine, and public health. Other areas of study include archaeology, biology, crime analysis, retail analysis, and many more. Much of the growth in this field has been fuelled by the availability of inexpensive high speed computing as well as large spatial and spatio-temporal datasets, and the development of sophisticated statistical tools within geographic information systems (Gelfand et al. 2010). Spatial statistics can also be found in other statistical applications such as MatLAB, R, and SAS.

Traditional GIS techniques include overlaying of layers, spatial queries, buffer analysis, and proximity calculations. Tools to perform 3D, raster, and network analysis are also included in traditional GIS applications. Spatial statistics are used for a variety of analyses, including pattern analysis, shape analysis, surface modelling and surface prediction, spatial regression, statistical comparisons of spatial datasets, statistical modelling, prediction of spatial interaction, etc.

Spatial statistics are used to access patterns, trends, and relationships to better understand geographic phenomena, suggest causes to explain geographic patterns, and make decisions with a high level of confidence. It is now possible to determine geographic patterns and distributions and determine whether they are statistically significant.

Within GIS, spatial statistics tools use area, length, proximity, orientation, or spatial relationships directly in their mathematics and can answer questions such as: Does the spatial pattern of a disease mirror the population at risk? Is there an unexpected spike in pharmaceutical purchases? Are new AIDS cases remaining geographically fixed? Spatial statistics tools within GIS that analyse patterns include: *Average nearest neighbour*, which calculates the average distance from every feature to its nearest neighbour based on feature centroids; *high/low clustering (Getis-Ord general G)*, which measures concentrations of high or low values for a study area; *spatial autocorrelation (global Moran's I)*, which measures clustering or dispersion based on feature locations and attribute values; *and multi-distance spatial cluster analysis (Ripley's K function)*, which assesses spatial clustering/dispersion for a set of geographic features over a range of distances. GIS tools that map clusters include *cluster and outlier analysis (Anselin's local Moran's I)* which, given a set of weighted features, identifies clusters of high or low values as well as spatial outliers; and *hot spot analysis (Getis-Ord Gi∗)* which, given a set of weighted features, identifies clusters of features with high values (hot spots) and clusters of features with low values (cold spots). There are also spatial statistics tools for modeling spatial relationships and performing spatial regression. Regression analysis may be used to model and explore spatial relationships. For example, regression analysis might explain why a particular disease rate is exceptionally high in a particular area of a region or country (Scott and Getis 2008) values (cold spots). There are also spatial statistics tools for modelling spatial relationships and performing spatial regression. Regression analysis may be used to model and explore spatial relationships. For example, regression analysis might explain why a particular disease rate is exceptionally high in a particular area of a region or country (Scott and Getis 2008).

Examples of spatial statistics can be found in many academic journals. One peer-reviewed scientific journal that provides a home for high quality work which straddles the areas of GIS, epidemiology, exposure science, and spatial statistics is *Spatial and Spatio-Temporal Epidemiology*. A recent article in this journal entitled 'A spatio-temporal model for estimating the long-term effects of air pollution on respiratory hospital admissions in Greater London' had five aims: (1) propose a new model for estimating the effects of air pollution on human health; (2) present a new study of the effects of air pollution for human health in London; (3) show that space–time models are needed to account for residual autocorrelation; (4) show that pollution is associated with significant increases in respiratory hospital admissions; and (5) provide fast and free supporting software written in the R language (Rushworth et al. 2014). Recently released publically available data of health and social statistics from National Cancer Institute's Surveillance Epidemiology and End Results (SEER, http://seer.cancer.gov/) database in the USA, and the Health and Social Care Information Centre (HSCIC, https://indicators.ic.nhs.uk/webview/) indicator portal in the UK, include population level annual aggregated summaries of disease incidence and socio-economic status for administrative units, such as electoral wards or census tracts. Additionally, modeled yearly average pollution concentrations estimated by computer dispersion models on a regular grid for the UK have also become freely available through the Department for the Environment, Food and Rural Affairs (DEFRA, http://uk-air.defra.gov.uk/data/pcm-data). These data sources have enabled researchers to estimate the long-term health impact of air pollution using small-area spatio-temporal study designs, which due to the easy availability of the data are quick and inexpensive to implement. While these studies cannot assess the causal health effects of air pollution due to their ecological design, their ease of implementation means that they contribute to and independently corroborate the body of evidence about the long-term population level impact of air pollution.

Discussion Task
Why is spatial statistics an important part of an epidemiological GIS study? Discuss

Conclusion

The first known GIS applications related to health were drawn using paper maps in the 1800s. Advances in aerial imagery and other technologies during wartime in the early twentieth century laid the foundation for GIS as we know it today. Early uses of GIS were government and land use and work done at the Harvard School of Design produced leaders in the GIS industry including today's largest GIS software vendor, Esri. The future of GIS is the integration of open source GIS, desktop, cloud based tools, and mobile devices. Social media and other means of collecting data offer new ways for public health officials to have a better understanding of communities. Organizations at all levels use GIS and advanced mapping technologies to better understand disease, the environment, and the overall health of the population world-wide. While there are advantages and disadvantages to GIS and maps, it is clear that advances in mapping applications and spatial statistics provide epidemiologists, medical doctors, scientists, and others in the field of public health tools to not only visualize, model, and share health related data, decisions can be made with solid scientific evidence.

References

Arnoff, S. (1995). *GIS: A management perspective* (pp. 48–50). Ottawa, CA: WDL.

Bolstad, P. (2008). *GIS fundamentals: A first text on geographic information systems* (3rd ed.). White Bear Lakem, MN: Eider Press.

Esri and Jack Dangermond. (2015). Retrieved from http://www.forbes.com/profile/jack-dangermond/

Esri customers. (2014). Retrieved from http://www.redlandsdailyfacts.com/social-affairs/20140531/redlands-tech-company-esri-aims-for-a-better-world.

Esri partners. (2013). Retrieved from http://techcrunch.com/2013/07/08/mapping-giant-esri-adds-real-time-traffic-information-from-nokias-here/

Esri storymaps. (2015). Retrieved from http://storymaps.arcgis.com/en/

Gelfand, A., Diggle, P., Guttorp, P., & Fuentes, M. (2010). *Handbook of spatial-statistics* (CRC handbooks of modern statistical methods). Boca Raton, FL: CRC Press (Preface).

Gettinger, D. (2014). *The Ultimate Way of Seeing: Aerial Photography in WWI, Center for the Study of the.* Bard College: Drone. Accessed January 28, 2014, from http://dronecenter.bard.edu/wwi-photography/.

Health and Human Services. (2005). Retrieved from http://www.hhs.gov/ocr/privacy/hipaa/understanding/coveredentities/De-identification/guidance.html#safeharborguidance

Healthcare Atlas. (2015). Retrieved from http://gis.oshpd.ca.gov/atlas.

Hoel, E, McGrath, M, & Gillgrass, C. (2009). *History of GIS in the computer automation era 1940 to 1969,* version 13. Esri User Conference San Diego, CA.

Koch, T. (2005). *Cartographies of disease: Maps, mapping, and medicine.* Redlands, CA: Esri Press.

Kurland, K., & Gorr, W. (2014). *GIS tutorial for health* (5th ed.). Redlands, CA: Esri Press.

Lubove, R. (1963). *The progressives and the slums: Tenement house reform in New York City.* Pittsburgh, PA: University of Pittsburgh Press. Appendix A.

Murak, J. (2013). *Regression analysis using GIS, MIT libraries.* Retrieved From https://libraries.mit.edu/files/gis/regression_presentation_iap2013.pdf.

National Cancer Institute. (2015). Retrieved from gis.cancer.gov

NYC DOHMH. (2015) Retrieved from http://www.nyc.gov/html/doh/html/data/gis-center.shtml.

Phillips, R. L., Jr., Kinman, E. L., Schnitzer, P. G., Lindbloom, E. J., & Ewigman, B. (2000). Using geographic information systems to understand health care access. *Archives of Family Medicine, 9*(10), 971–978.

QGIS. (2015). Retrieved from http://www.qgis.org/en/site/

Reichhardt, T. (2006). *Air and Space Magazine, website.* http://www.airspacemag.com/space/the-first-photo-from-space-13721411.

Rushworth, A., Lee, D., & Mitchell, R. (2014). A spatio-temporal model for estimating the long-term effects of air pollution on respiratory hospital admissions in Greater London. *Spatial and Spatio-temporal Epidemiology, 10,* 29–38.

Sampson, D. (2014). *URISA, website.* http://www.urisa.org/awards/roger-tomlinson/.

Scott, L., & Getis, A. (2008). Spatial statistics. In K. Kemp (Ed.), *Encyclopedia of geographic informations*. Thousand Oaks, CA: Sage.

Syed, S., Gerber, B., & Sharp, L. (2013). Traveling towards disease: Transportation barriers to health care access. *Journal of Community Health, 38*(5), 976–993.

Univac, I. (2015). US Census website. Retrieved from https://www.census.gov/history/www/innovations/technology/univac_i.html.

US Census. (2015). Retrieved from http://www.census.gov/population/international/

Vinten-Johansen, P., Brody, H., Paneth, N., Rachman, S., Rip, M., & Zuck, D. (2003). *Cholera, chloroform, and the science of medicine: A life of John Snow*. New York: Oxford University Press.

World Health Organization. (2015). Maps and spatial information technologies (Geographical Information Systems) in health and environment decision-making. Retrieved from http://www.who.int/heli/tools/maps/en/

Recommended Reading

Rushworth, A., Lee, D., & Mitchell, R. (2014). A spatio-temporal model for estimating the long-term effects of air pollution on respiratory hospital admissions in Greater London. *Spatial and Spatio-temporal Epidemiology, 10*, 29–38.

Koch, T. (2005). *Cartographies of disease: Maps, mapping, and medicine*. Redlands, CA: Esri Press.

Synthesising Public Health Evidence

Ivan Gee and Krishna Regmi

Abstract Public Health research is multi-disciplinary, complex and tries to understand problems in a 'real-world' context and this can make it hard to apply to practice and services that aim to improve health outcomes. Increasingly it has been realised that the mass of health evidence generated needs to be synthesised effectively. This chapter will explore the growing focus on this issue, the tools developed to synthesis evidence well and examples of evidence synthesis in practice.

After reading this chapter you will be able to:

- Define the meaning of research and research process
- Understand the need for public health evidence synthesis
- Describe the tools and techniques used to synthesise evidence effectively

Before we can start to synthesise evidence we need to have some understanding of what evidence is and where the new evidence being explored comes from. Fundamentally as Lomas et al. (2005, p. 1) suggest 'evidence concerns facts (actual or asserted) intended for use in support of a conclusion.' Decision makers tend to view evidence colloquially, that is evidence is anything that can give a reason for believing something relevant is considered evidence. Researchers will tend to view evidence scientifically, it must be produced by robust, systematic and replicable methods that are clearly defined. So evidence is something that can be used to support a conclusion, but it is not the same as a conclusion (Lomas et al. 2005). Evidence can, and should, support decision making but the collection of evidence alone is not going to make the decisions.

Evidence for Public Health impacts and interventions is generated through the process of research. Research is about generating new information, doing some-

I. Gee (✉)
Center for Public Health, Liverpool John Moores University,
Henry Cotton Building, 15-21 Webster St., Liverpool L3 2ET, UK
e-mail: i.l.gee@ljmu.ac.uk

K. Regmi
Faculty of Health and Social Sciences, University of Bedfordshire,
Putteridge Bury Campus, IHR-32, Luton LU2 8LE, UK

© Springer International Publishing Switzerland 2016   129
K. Regmi, I. Gee (eds.), *Public Health Intelligence*,
DOI 10.1007/978-3-319-28326-5_7

thing new, collecting information to answer specific research questions and testing ideas or hypotheses.

There are several characteristics of good research. It should be:

- **Systematic:** there is an agreed system for performing observations and measurement
- **Rigorous:** the agreed system is followed exactly.
- **Reproducible:** all the techniques, apparatus and materials used in making observations and measurements are written down in enough detail to allow other to reproduce the same process.
- **Repeatable:** researchers often repeat their observations and measurements several times in order to increase the reliability of the data. (Bruce et al. 2008)

Types of Research

Research is typically divided into quantitative or qualitative methods but these are not mutually exclusive and should be seen as complementary approaches to obtaining evidence. Creswell (2014) has described these two approaches as being on a continuum, with quantitative methods *tending* to explore issues through numbers, and qualitative methods *tending* to examine issues through words. Using this research typology (or classification), this would only distinguish questions which seek to measure something (quantitative) from those that don't (qualitative). This seems to be only a small element of the range of research questions that social scientists address. You might have already noticed that qualitative research doesn't seek to measure anything … but may do much more, whilst quantitative research does seek to measure … but may also do much more. A third type of research is termed mixed methods research, where researchers would combine both qualitative and quantitative methods (Creswell 2014). We can see this range of approaches in evidence syntheses as well as in the primary research.

> **So we can summarise research into three main approaches:**
> - Quantitative
> - Qualitative
> - Mixed-methods (Using both quantitative and qualitative methods)

Although these can be viewed as the main divisions they can be subdivided into many more specific categories. For example, a working paper for the National Centre for Research Methods categorised research designs into 20 types (Beissel-Durrant 2004).

Types of Research Questions

We will now focus more on the types of questions that one needs to think about. Research questions should always relate to the nature of the problem being explored. If you look at any research proposal or research article, they will tend to have clearly stated aim(s), objectives and/or specific research questions.

Discussion Task
Search for research papers on a public health topic, such as alcohol consumption, levels of inactivity etc. How do researchers frame their aims or research questions?

Comments: You will notice that there are 4–5 main types of questions.

Some research questions (outcome) relate to describing things within contextual paradigms (descriptions of type of research), some relate to comparing one aspect to another (comparisons), others are related to measurements, giving/emphasising values or determining some relationships between or amongst different attributes.

All of these approaches can form the framework for evidence synthesis and individual studies using these approaches can contribute to the evidence being synthesised.

Research Synthesis

Within this section we will try to define the meaning of research synthesis, its importance, and how to synthesise diverse sources of evidence. It is important that policy-makers and managers always use a wide range of sources of evidence in making decisions about policy and the organisation of services. However, they are under increasing pressure to adopt a more systematic approach to the utilisation of the complex evidence base in healthcare. Sometimes, decision-makers must address some complicated questions about the nature and significance of the problem to be addressed; the nature of proposed interventions; their varying impact; cost-effectiveness; acceptability and so on (Mays et al. 2005).

As Coast (2006) notes, the meaning and purpose of synthesising research is identifying

- What is known from what has been done?

NOT

- What has been done?

Why Do We Need Evidence Synthesis?

A quick perusal of public health research journals will rapidly show the huge variety of research evidence generated to help us understand public health problems. Firstly the subject is very multidisciplinary, evidence is generated by a wide range of disciplines including:

- Biostatistics
- Epidemiology
- Environmental health
- Global health
- Health education
- Health improvement/promotion
- Health protection
- Occupational health

Furthermore health is a broad concept and many different factors influence our health. All these are studied and explored in increasing volume and depth e.g:

- Alcohol
- Communicable diseases
- Drugs
- Mental health
- Obesity
- Sexual health
- Exercise
- Tobacco

To focus on just one example consider a case study for evidence around heart disease, our largest cause of death.

Case Study: Heart Disease Research

Heart disease is our largest cause of death and numerous research has been conducted to try and understand how heart disease progresses, what factors increase the risk of developing heart disease and how effective interventions are at preventing its development? Conduct a simple web search (e.g. using Google Scholar) for academic research articles on these three topics:

1. Aetiology of heart disease (how it progresses)
2. Risk factors for heart disease
3. Interventions for heart disease

Comments: you will find your searches yield huge numbers, millions of papers. Also within these topics there is great variety e.g. for risk factors, research might have explored factors such as:

- Age
- Hypertension (high blood pressure)

(continued)

(continued)
- Cholesterol
- Diabetes
- Smoking
- Alcohol
- Diet
- Cocaine
- Obesity
- Exercise
- Preeclampsia
- Family history

and there are many others (NHLBI 2015), so there is a need to synthesise all this evidence.

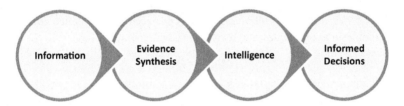

Fig. 1 Transforming information into informed decisions

Keeping track of all this evidence is clearly a challenge. Public health decision makers can be overwhelmed by the volume of data and evidence, i.e. by too much information. Increasingly public health organisations and researchers have been developing tools and techniques to help synthesise the evidence, transforming the mass of information in to useful intelligence, so that we can make decisions based on clear and accurate summaries of the range of evidence available (Fig. 1).

Research synthesis is important in public health because it allows researchers to view problems from multiple perspectives, contextualise information, develop a more complete understanding of a problem, triangulate results, quantify hard-to-measure constructs, provide illustrations of the context for trends, examine processes/experiences along with outcomes, and capture a macro picture of a health system (Creswell and Clark 2011). We can argue that balanced inference on best available evidence is always important, not a detailed description of everything on the subject. It is equally important to note that chosen approaches or methods should be rigorous, using 'scientific' methodology in terms of being replicable/account-able/having updateable findings, minimising biases and errors, as well as being appropriate to answer the focussed question(s).

Discussion Task

Read the definition of research synthesis first: Research synthesis can be considered as an approach of integrating/synthesising several studies' attributes, i.e. study design, findings and quality; not only to be able to identify research gaps or 'silences' that require new primary studies, but also to provide a unique presentation of multiple realities or truths (see Mosteller and Colditz 1996, p. 4; Pope and Mays 2006).

Identify four or five important purposes and consider how this concept relates to making appropriate design in public health or health policy.

Types, Methods and Approaches to Research Synthesis

As Popay and Roberts (2006, p. 1) note 'since the early 1990s the *science* of evidence review and synthesis has had a growth spurt and has developed rapidly.' There are now well established tools and methodologies to support effective research synthesis, an example being the international Cochrane collaboration, which publishes evidence synthesis as well as providing best practice guidance on methodologies and online training materials (Cochrane 2015).

Research synthesis is a comprehensive review that looks for, and evaluates, existing research evidence, rather than a traditional literature review. It is interesting to note that methods of synthesis that can accommodate diversity both of questions and of evidence are needed. For example, policy-makers seeking to understand barriers to access to healthcare will need to draw on qualitative evidence (for example, generated through ethnographies and interview studies of help-seeking behaviour) as well as quantitative evidence (perhaps generated through studies of rates of referral). Excluding any type of evidence on grounds of its methodology could have potentially detrimental consequences (Mays et al. 2005, p. 45). There is no single, agreed framework or method for synthesising such diverse forms of evidence, and many of the approaches potentially applicable to such an endeavour were devised for either qualitative or quantitative synthesis and/or for analysing primary data.

Traditional literature reviews can be limited by bias in the selection of information, driven by researcher bias, limited search strategies, and lack of access to resources. Digitisation of resources and the ubiquitous access to computer based search engines have eliminated some of these problems and the systematisation of reviews means we can summarise evidence in a less biased manner.

Mays et al. (2005) identify four basic approaches:

- Narrative (including traditional 'literature reviews' and more methodologically explicit approaches such as 'thematic analysis', 'narrative synthesis', 'realist synthesis' and 'meta-narrative mapping')

- Quantitative (which either use data from quantitative sources only or convert all evidence into quantitative form using techniques such as 'quantitative case survey' or 'content analysis')
- Qualitative (which convert all available evidence into qualitative form using techniques such as 'meta-ethnography' and 'qualitative cross-case analysis'),
- Bayesian meta-analysis and decision analysis (which can convert qualitative evidence such as preferences about different outcomes into quantitative form or 'weights' to use in quantitative synthesis).

The choice of approach or method will be determined by the purpose of the review and the nature of the available evidence. Often more than one approach or method will be required to make the evidence credible and dependable.

As Sheldon (2005) warns, we need to be aware of the following points while assessing and synthesising any research evidence:

- Low statistical power—studies may be small and in themselves insufficient to be able to provide reliable evidence of benefit or harm. This increases the risk of false negatives.
- Researcher/expert bias—different researchers will favour certain conclusions and may give different weights to the same evidence and write up their results with a different spin
- Contextual variability—there may be reasons to think that contextual factors are likely to affect the impact of an intervention, so policy which is effective in one context may not be so in another
- Methodological and theoretical incompleteness—the reliability of the evidence is likely to be greater if studies of different designs are examined and are mutually supportive. Studies approaching the same problem from different theoretical perspectives can also be illuminating
- Policy relevance—Policy decisions often need information not only on whether an intervention works but also on the factors that influence how well it works, whether these can be modified, and the distribution of the benefits and costs. It is most unlikely that any one study will cover all these issues.

So how do we go about conducting a research synthesis? We will explore these separately for quantitative and qualitative as these different research approaches also result in some differences in synthesis methods.

Quantitative Synthesis: Systematic Reviews and Meta-analysis

A casual analysis of daily newspapers will identify health stories based on single quantitative research studies e.g. extolling the benefits of moderate consumption of red wine. A few months' later readers might view another story, based on a different study, which has identified risks associated with moderate alcohol consumption. It's not surprising that the public and policy makers alike are confused. Systematic

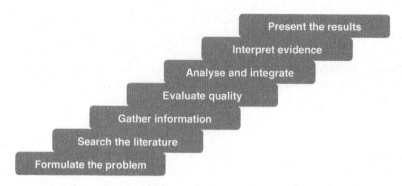

Fig. 2 The seven steps in a systematic review

reviews attempt to avoid the difficulties of relying on single studies, which can often be misrepresented or 'cherry picked' in this way. They combine information from multiple sources in a clear and systematic process that tries to minimise any bias in selection of studies. Systematic reviews, assess, select and combine the findings of the selected studies to identify common conclusions. There are commonly seven steps in a systematic evidence synthesis or systematic review (Cooper 2010) (Fig. 2):

Step 1: Formulating the problem—in any research synthesis the first step is always to identify what are the concepts that are to be studied? What is the hypothesis to be tested, or what research questions will be explored?

Step 2: Searching the literature—this should be systematic in nature. So clear search criteria are established that address the aim(s) of the study. There is a defined strategy for identifying literature from a range of sources that includes published journal articles, reports and grey literature and unpublished material. A great deal of time and effort in systematic research synthesis goes into ensuring that the literature search is comprehensive.

Step 3: Gathering information from studies—this involves extracting the information from each study that is relevant to the synthesis aim(s). Not all information in each identified study might be relevant to the aims of the synthesis. Typically, due to the limitations of electronic search engines, the majority of studies identified in the literature review are rejected at this point as not being directly relevant to the synthesis. Again clear criteria need to be established to identify what information is to be extracted in order to ensure this is done systematically and without bias.

Step 4: Evaluating the quality of studies—once data are extracted the researcher(s) make critical judgements about the data quality for each study. This will be informed by factors such as the clarity of the study methodology reporting, or the type of study (e.g. case control or randomised controlled trial). Clearly if this step is not conduced in a fair and systematic way it can be a major source of bias and lead to criticism of the synthesis.

Step 5: Analysing and integrating the outcomes of studies—in this step the data from each individual study is integrated with the other studies. In systematic reviews this might be a process of identifying common findings between different studies and exploring those collectively. Within quantitative synthesis this can be taken a step further by using a **meta-analysis** (or metanalysis). A meta-analysis will take the statistical data from each selected study and combine these to provide pooled data that can then be statistically analysed. The advantage of meta-analysis is to provide a much larger effective sample size and to reduce statistical uncertainty.

Step 6: Interpreting the evidence—as with any study the researcher needs to interpret the evidence provided by the study and identity clear conclusions from the synthesis.

Step 7: Presenting the results—for the synthesis to be useful the results must be presented effectively. Of particular importance within research synthesis is to clearly communicate how the synthesis was conducted i.e. how the first six steps were performed.

An example of the results from a quantitative meta-analysis is shown in Fig. 3. This is a typical type of plot used in metanalysis studies called a Forest Plot.

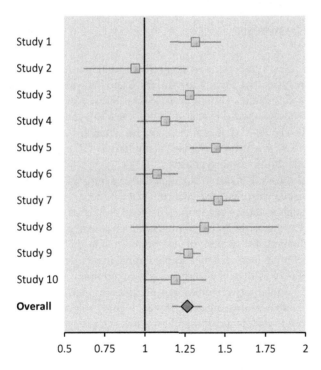

Fig. 3 An example Forest plot showing odds ratios for ten studies and the pooled overall estimate when the individual studies are combined. (*Source*: Neyeloff et al. 2012)

Discussion Task
Examine Fig. 3. Imagine this is showing results from ten studies on tobacco smoke exposure of householders and the odds of their developing lung cancer. What does this tell you about the power of applying meta-analysis and pooling data from multiple studies?

Comments: The plot shows odds ratios and the 95% confidence intervals for each study. There is considerable variation in the estimates and in the levels of confidence. Some studies have odds ratios, and confidence intervals that are >1.0 (i.e. no difference between those exposed and those not exposed to tobacco smoke) e.g. Study 1. These suggest that lung cancer is more likely in those exposed at home. But other studies have odds ratios that are < 1.0 (e.g. Study 2) or confidence intervals that span 1.0 e.g. Study 4 and for these we cannot be sure there is any difference in lung cancer risk between the exposed and not-exposed. However, when all ten studies are combined we see an increase in our confidence of the estimate, so the method has allowed us to move from some uncertainty due to conflicting estimates from different studies to an overall prediction.

Qualitative Synthesis

Qualitative evidence synthesis is an umbrella term increasingly used to describe a group of review types that attempt to synthesise and analyse findings from primary qualitative research studies (Booth et al. 2011). Some researchers have criticised qualitative synthesis suggesting that it is not valid to synthesise non-quantifiable data. Booth (2001) on the other hand has suggested that this can be viewed as 'insidious discrimination' via 'institutionalised quantitativism'. So are qualitative research (data) appropriate for research synthesis?

At one level this is difficult to say, qualitative synthesis are unlikely to use the sort of randomised controlled study designs that that been the mainstay of quantitative synthesis such as those seen in the Cochrane collection. It is also less likely to have been used as the methodology for intervention research so it will tend not to be useful for evaluating the success of interventions. On the other hand qualitative synthesis is becoming increasingly accepted as having a role in the systematic evaluation of qualitative evidence. Clearly people are complex and not always rational organisms and so qualitative studies can provide us with information that is not amenable to quantitative investigation. If we are going to make use of this information then methods to systematically synthesise this evidence are needed. Increasingly well-established organisations such as the Cochrane collaboration are incorporating qualitative synthesis. Since 2012 the Cochrane collaboration has had a qualitative and implementation methods group that provides resources and training on the use of qualitative synthesis methods.

As with quantitative synthesis we can utilise the same seven steps of synthesising evidence which were mentioned earlier and shown in Fig. 2:

1. Formulating the problem
2. Searching the literature
3. Gathering information from studies
4. Evaluating the quality of studies
5. Analysing and integrating the outcomes of studies
6. Interpreting the evidence
7. Presenting the results

Most of these steps require similar processes for quantitative and qualitative synthesis. However in qualitative synthesis searching the literature can be more problematical. Qualitative research tends to be less well indexed than quantitative research, although this is improving. It is also often found in smaller and less well circulated journals, making obtaining individual articles more difficult and time consuming. Evaluating the quality of the studies will also require different criteria, e.g. the size of the study (in terms of numbers of participants) is less important in qualitative research.

One of the complexities when trying to understand qualitative synthesis is the plethora of methods that have been developed in comparison to quantitative synthesis. Figure 4 shows the variety of methods that have been proposed and a selection of these are discussed below.

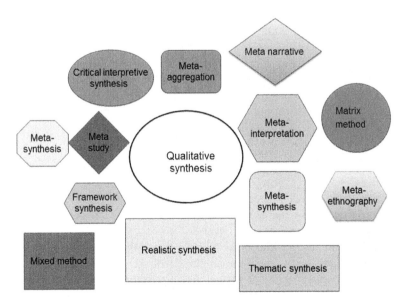

Fig. 4 Qualitative synthesis methodologies

Meta-ethnography

Meta-ethnography was proposed as an alternative to meta-analysis by Noblit and Hare (1988), whereby synthesis is about bringing separate parts together into a whole. It is viewed as a synergistic process so the result of the synthesis is greater than sum of the parts. There are several tools used within meta-ethnography to conduct the synthesis. (1) Reciprocal translational analysis (RTA) requires the 'translation' of ideas and concepts between individual studies to identify underlying concepts that are common to the individual studies. (2) Refutational synthesis examines contradictions between individual studies. The synthesis must then take into account the competing explanations. (3) Lines-of-argument (LOA) synthesis involves building up an overall picture of the whole (e.g. organisation, community, culture, etc.) from studies of its separate parts.

Grounded Theory

Grounded theory is a common methodological approach for individual qualitative research studies, but it has also been applied as a technique for qualitative synthesis. The general processes within a grounded theory approach include: simultaneous data collection and analysis; an inductive approach to analysis i.e. allowing theory to emerge from the data; use of the constant comparison method; use of theoretical sampling to reach theoretical saturation; and importantly, the generation of new theory (Barnet-Page and Thomas. 2009). The majority of applications of grounded theory synthesis (Eaves 2001; Kearney 1988 have used the approach because it matches 'like with like', i.e. they have used individual papers based on grounded theory approaches to generate a grounded theory synthesis. This is in contrast to meta-ethnography synthesis which seeks to integrate qualitative studies that might have used different theoretical approaches into a single synthesis.

Thematic Synthesis

The aim of thematic synthesis is to combine the approaches used in meta-ethnography and grounded theory (Thomas and Harden 2008). It was developed in order to produce reviews that are able to explore intervention need, appropriateness and acceptability, as well as effectiveness. People's views and experiences are taken into account and hypotheses are then developed that can be tested against the findings of qualitative studies. There are three main steps to a thematic synthesis: (1) Free line-by-line coding of textual findings from the primary studies; (2) Organisation of the free codes into 'descriptive' themes; and (3) Generation of 'analytical' themes, using the descriptive themes the analysis develops a new interpretation which goes beyond the original studies.

Textual Narrative Synthesis

This is an approach which takes individual studies and organises them into more homogenous groups. Typically the characteristics of the studies, their context, quality and types of findings are reported using a standard format and then the scope, similarities and differences are compared across studies in order to generate overall conclusions from the data i.e. the synthesis. The technique has been particularly successful in synthesising different types of research evidence e.g. qualitative, quantitative and economic studies. In their comparison of textual narrative synthesis with thematic synthesis (Lucas et al. 2007) found that textual narrative synthesis is valuable for generating future research hypotheses as it is particularly good at identifying gaps in the evidence.

Meta-study

This is a multi-faceted approach to synthesis with three components of analysis that are conducted before the synthesis: (1) Meta-data-analysis (the analysis of findings). This is similar to meta-ethnography as it is interpretive, looking to identify the similarities and differences between study accounts; (2) Meta-method (the analysis of methods) examines the methodologies used by individual studies e.g. issues of sampling, data collection, research design etc. This is similar to the procedure of critical appraisal frequently used in quantitative synthesis; and, (3) Meta-theory (the analysis of theory). This involves exploration theoretical assumptions of the different studies included in the synthesis. Meta-synthesis is then required to 'bring back together ideas that have been taken apart' and create a new interpretation of the phenomenon under investigation (Ring et al. 2011).

Meta-narrative

Greenhalgh et al. (2005) developed the meta-narrative approach in order to synthesise evidence that would then inform policy-making. Their work was around the diffusion of innovations in health service delivery and organisation, where there was a need to synthesise findings from studies based on different theories and that utilised different study designs. They identified different research 'traditions' and sampled studies from each of these. Key features of each tradition were then mapped (e.g. historical roots, scope, theoretical basis; research questions; instruments used; main findings; historical development of the body of knowledge; and strengths and limitations). This exercise generated maps of 13 'meta-narratives' from which seven key dimensions (themes) were synthesised. The approach is relatively new and not yet fully established but offers the potential to examine and synthesise policy-relevant research, such as exploring the success or failure of complex health interventions.

Critical Interpretive Synthesis

Critical interpretive synthesis (CIS) is an adaptation of meta-ethnography and grounded theory techniques. It was developed by Dixon-woods et al. (2006) as they needed to adapt traditional meta-ethnographic methods for synthesis of both quantitative and qualitative data. Dixon-woods et al. (2006) suggest two key features of CIS distinguishes it from conventional systematic review methods (1) it rejects the stage approach to review. Processes of question formulation, searching, selection, data extraction, critique and synthesis are characterised as iterative, interactive, dynamic and recursive rather than as fixed procedures to be accomplished in a pre-defined sequence; and (2) there is an explicit orientation towards theory generation in CIS.

Framework Synthesis

Framework synthesis is based on framework analysis. It is based on the observation that qualitative research produces very large amounts of textual data in the form of transcripts, fieldnotes etc. and that this volume of information presents a challenge for rigorous analysis. To overcome this framework synthesis takes a highly structured approach to organising and analysing the data that has a quantitative 'feel' and a deductive approach. It uses a pre-defined 'framework' for the analysis rather than developing themes etc. directly from the data. In addition it typically involves numerical index codes and rearranging data into charts etc.

Discussion Task
Look at Fig. 4 and choose 2–3 specific methods for qualitative synthesis. Explore the literature to identify individual studies that have used these methods in a topic that interests you and consider the following:

- What was the approach and why was it used for this topic?
- What information was gained from this approach that would not have been obtainable from a quantitative synthesis?
- What is the potential relevance for public health/public health intelligence?

Selection of Qualitative Synthesis Method

One of the difficulties with qualitative synthesis, as with qualitative research is the large and increasing number of alternative approaches, which is why Fig. 4 portrays the methods as a Pandora's Box (there are wonderful things inside, but some risk in letting them all out!). As we have shown in the previous summaries the various synthesis methods all approach collection, review, analysis and synthesis differently. Some of the differences are modest e.g. Critical Interpretive Synthesis shares many attributes of meta-ethnography, and some are more substantial, e.g. Framework synthesis is deductive (testing theory using analysis of the data) whereas all the other approaches are inductive (inducing the conclusions and new theory from the data). There is no 'correct' approach to take and many more experienced researchers often tend to stick to the familiar, ignoring the Pandora's Box of alternatives. Ideally though, we should choose a suitable method based on the purpose of the research, the type of studies that will be examined and the nature of the data that they have produced. But other factors such as the timeframe for the synthesis, resources available, researcher expertise and the audience for the synthesis will also inevitably to be taken into account.

Discussion Task

Though we highlighted some strengths, some questions (adopted from Mays et al. 2005) are still unanswered. You should consider these, for example:

- Is it always acceptable to synthesise studies?
- Is it feasible to synthesize disparate evidence?
- Should reviews start with a well-defined question and how many papers are required?

Conclusion

This chapter has sought to explore the nature of research evidence and how this is synthesised using different synthesis approaches. We have seen that both quantitative and qualitative approaches to synthesis are both possible and valuable. These should be seen as complementary rather than competing, and all feeding into the process of transforming raw data into information and then intelligence that can be used for the development of public health policy and practice. The different synthesis methods are very varied and the choice of method will depend upon whether concepts and theories are clear in advance, the purpose of the work, whether they are generating, exploring or testing theory or advancing understanding; to inform the choice of interventions, or to inform the development and implementation of interventions; and whether data is qualitative, quantitative or mixed.

144 I. Gee and K. Regmi

References

Booth, A. (2001). Cochrane or cock-eyed? How should we conduct systematic reviews of qualitative research? *In Qualitative Evidence-Based Practice Conference, May 14–16, 2001, Coventry University.*
Booth, A., Papaioannou, D., & Sutton, A. (2011). *Systematic approaches to a successful literature review*. London: Sage.
Barnet-Page, E., & Thomas, J. (2009). *Methods for the synthesis of qualitative research: A critical review*. ESRC National Centre for Research Methods, NCRM Working Paper Series Number (01/09).
Beissel-Durrant, G. (2004). *A typology of research methods within the social sciences*. National Centre for Research Methods (NCRM) Working Paper.
Bruce, N., Pope, D., & Stanistreet, D. (2008). *Quantitative methods for health research: A practical interactive guide to epidemiology and statistics*. Oxford, England: Wiley.
Coast, E. (2006). *Qualitative research synthesis: What, why and how? Institut Superieur des Sciences de la Population*. Burkina Faso: University of Ouagadougou.
Cochrane. (2015). *The Cochrane collection*. Retrieved September 18, 2015, from http://uk.cochrane.org/.
Cooper, H. (2010). *Research synthesis and meta-analysis a step-by-step approach*. London: Sage.
Creswell, J. W., & Clark, V. L. (2011). *Designing and conducting mixed methods research*. London: Sage.
Creswell, J. W. (2014). *Research design: Qualitative, quantitative, and mixed methods approaches*. London: Sage.
Dixon-woods, M., Cavers, D., Agarwal, S., Annandale, E., Arthur, A., Harvey, J., et al. (2006). Conducting critical interpretative synthesis of the literature on access to healthcare by vulnerable groups. *BMC Research Methodology, 6*, 35.
Eaves, Y. D. (2001). A synthesis technique for grounded theory data analysis. *Journal of Advanced Nursing, 35*, 654–663.
Greenhalgh, T., Robert, G., Macfarlane, F., Bate, S. P., Kyriakidou, O., & Peacock, R. (2005). Storylines of research in diffusion of innovation: A meta-narrative approach to systematic review. *Social Science and Medicine, 61*(2), 417–430.
Kearney, M. H. (1988). Ready-to-wear: Discovering grounded formal theory. *Research on Nursing and Health, 21*, 179–186.
Lomas, L., Culyer, T., McCutcheon, C., McAuley, L., & Law, S. (2005). *Conceptualizing and combining evidence for health system guidance*. Ottawa, ON, Canada: Canadian Health Services Research Foundation.
Lucas, P.J., Baird, J., Arai, L., Law, C., & Roberts, H.M. (2007). Worked examples of alternative methods for the synthesis of qualitative and quantitative research in systematic reviews. *BMC Medical Research Methodology,7*(4), doi:10.1186/1471-2288-7-4.
Mays, N., Pope, C., & Popay, J. (2005). Systematically reviewing qualitative and quantitative evidence to inform management and policy-making in the health field. *Journal of Health Services Research and Policy, 10*(Suppl 1), 6–20.
Mosteller, F., & Colditz, G. A. (1996). Understanding research synthesis (meta-analysis). *Annual Review of Public Health, 17*, 1–23. doi:10.1146/annurev.pu.17.050196.000245.
Neyeloff, J., Fuchs, S. C., & Moreira, L. B. (2012). Meta-analyses and Forest plots using a microsoft excel spreadsheet: step-by-step guide focusing on descriptive data analysis. *BMC Research, 5*, 52. doi:10.1186/1756-0500-5-52.
NHLBI. (2015). *What are the risk factors for heart disease?* [Online]. National Heart Lung and Blood Institute. Retrieved July 15, 2015, from http://www.nhlbi.nih.gov/health/educational/hearttruth/lower-risk/risk-factors.htm.

Noblit, G., & Hare, R. (1988). *Meta-ethnography: Synthesing qualitative studies*. Newbury Park, CA: Sage.

Popay, J., & Roberts, H. (2006). Introduction: Methodological issues in the synthesis of diverse sources of evidence. In J. Popay (Ed.), *Moving beyond effectiveness in evidence synthesis methodological issues in the synthesis of diverse sources of evidence*. London: NICE.

Pope, C., & Mays, N. (2006). Qualitative research in healthcare. In C. Pope & N. Mays (Eds.), *Synthesising qualitative research* (pp. 142–152). London: Sage.

Ring, N., Ritchie, K., Mandava, L., & Jepson, R. (2011). *A guide to synthesising qualitative research for researchers undertaking health technology assessments and systematic reviews*. Edinburgh, Scotland: NHS Quality Improvement.

Sheldon, T. A. (2005). Making evidence synthesis more useful for management and policy-making. Journal of Health Services Research and Policy, 10(Suppl 1), 1–5. doi:10.1258/1355819054308521.

Thomas, J., & Harden, A. (2008). Methods for the thematic synthesis of qualitative research in systematic reviews. *BMC Medical Research Methodology, 8*, 45.

Recommended Reading

Jackson, N., Waters, E., & The Guidelines for Systematic Reviews of Health Promotion and Public Health Interventions Taskforce. (2004). The challenges of systematically reviewing public health interventions. *Journal of Public Health, 26*(3), 303–307.

Lavis, J. N., Oxman, A. D., Lewin, S., & Fretheim, A. (2009). SUPPORT Tools for evidence-informed health Policymaking (STP). *Health Research Policy and Systems, 7*(Supp 1), I1.

Pope, C., Mays, N., & Popay, J. (2007). *Synthesising qualitative and quantitative health evidence*. London: Sage.

Sandelowski, M., & Barroso, J. (2007). *Handbook of synthesising qualitative research*. New York: Springer.

Policy Formulation, Planning, and Evaluation

Colin Thunhurst

Abstract This chapter will address the processes and intelligence needs of formulating policy and planning and evaluating interventions for the attainment of public health objectives. It will adopt and introduce you to the Whole Systems perspective on public health issues and the complexity of interventions resulting from the adoption of such a perspective. It will introduce methods of Public Health Systems Analysis and indicate their key role in formulating interventions which operationalise a Whole Systems perspective. It will show how these can be integrated into a planning spiral, through use of a Logical Framework, highlighting the information needs. It will consider the critical issue of the monitoring and evaluation of complex public health interventions. And it will highlight the Public Health Intelligence needs of Whole Systems Public Health.

After reading this chapter you will be able to:

- Understand the importance and distinctive features of adopting a Whole Systems Approach to Public Health
- Appreciate the value of appropriate analytic tools compatible with such an approach
- Recognise the need to put community involvement at the centre of such an approach
- Operate a planning cycle/spiral according to conventional stages within it
- Construct a logical framework and recognise the value of its use for the design, monitoring and evaluation of complex public health interventions

C. Thunhurst (✉)
Faculty of Health and Life Sciences, Coventry University, Stone Cottage,
5 Aire View, Coventry, Keighley, West Yorkshire BD20 5LH, UK
e-mail: colinthunhurst@outlook.com

© Springer International Publishing Switzerland 2016
K. Regmi, I. Gee (eds.), *Public Health Intelligence*,
DOI 10.1007/978-3-319-28326-5_8

Introduction

In the chapter that follows, we will look at the processes of formulating public health policy and planning and evaluating meaningful public health interventions for the achievement of public health objectives. In particular, we will identify and isolate the public health intelligence needs of the policy formation and planning processes. Broadly, we will equate policy formation with the production of public health programmes and planning with the production of public health projects— the latter constituting the actual point of implementing an intervention. Although the respective stages of these processes will be presented sequentially, it is important to stress from the outset that they are not separate activities. In the real world of public health it will be necessary to iterate, both within and between, the respective processes. In this way, central or 'macro' policy formation will not become isolated from or ignorant of implementation on the ground. To begin with it is important that all actors, from policy formers to on-the-ground implementers, share a common view of the need for an integrated vision of the determinants of public health outcomes.

Public Health Policy Formation

The Whole Systems Approach

Over recent decades Public Health has moved hesitatingly towards a better under-standing of the complexity of the multiple influences that determine health out-comes and which must be addressed if Public Health interventions are to achieve their intended impact. This greater awareness has emerged to a certain degree out of a sense of disappointment at the limited success or unintended consequences of implementing simple 'mono-causal' interventions. Health education programmes which failed to address the social and economic context of participants have, for example, proved to have a differential impact on communities and thereby contrib-uted to an increase in social inequalities in smoking and smoking-related ill-health.

Alongside, (and to a degree because of), the practical demonstration of the lim-ited value of one-dimensional public health thinking there has been a paradigm shift in public health understanding. This paradigm shift has been reviewed more thor-oughly elsewhere (Thunhurst 2012). Within the UK and elsewhere within the devel-oped world the paradigm shift was sparked by a realisation of the apparent failure of respective health care systems to tackle persisting inequalities in health outcomes. This produced the layered representations of health determinants most usually asso-ciated with the work of Dahlgren and Whitehead (1991) which has been central to public health for the last three decades and which has provided the inner core for more developed representations, such as the 'health map' of Barton and Grant

(2006). It pre-dated the more dynamic representations of disease aetiology incorpo-rated into the *Life Course Approach* (Kuh and Ben-Shlomo 2004). Consciously or unconsciously, the advance in thinking taking place in developing countries mir-rored those which had driven health policy in developing countries since the 1970s. Specifically, the *Primary Health Care Approach*, formulated out of the Alma Ata Conference in 1977, had stressed the need for comprehensive interventions that tackled underlying social and economic determinants as well as their 'front-line' manifestations in health outcomes (Thunhurst 2012, 2013).

It was perhaps then not unsurprising that the most concerted attempt to coalesce the respective paradigmatic threads into an integrated paradigm, the *Whole Systems Approach*, was sparked by a global WHO initiative, the Commission on Social Determinants of Health (WHO 2008). This was led by Sir Michael Marmot who drew this approach into a subsequent review that his team at University College London undertook into health inequality in the UK (Marmot 2010).

As with all paradigm shifts, advances in theoretical articulation are generally predicated upon practical considerations. Thus it was, for example, that the Foresight Report (Butland et al. 2007) on tackling obesity in the UK had pre-figured the Marmot Review of health inequalities by adopting an analysis of the determinants of obesity which comprehensively spanned 'societal influences', 'food production', the 'activity environment' as well as 'individual psychology', 'food consumption', 'individual activity' and 'biology'. Also pre-empting the soon-to-be-published Marmot Review, a NICHE scoping study on preventing obesity using a 'whole-system' approach (NICHE 2010) contained the following succinct encapsulation:

> 'For the purpose of this guidance, a 'whole-system' sustainable approach to obesity involves a broad set of integrated policies combined with population-wide and targeted measures. This includes action by central and local government, industry, communities, families and society as a whole. It also involves shifting attention away from individual risk factors or isolated interventions and considering many influences simultaneously, ...'. (NICHE 2010, p. 2)

Although the perceived intractability of obesity has been the most prominent focus of the new public health thinking, applicability to other fields of social policy is increasing. Friel et al. (2015, p. 1) 'illustrate the pathways between trade and health, and explore the emerging ... policy landscape and its implications for health and health equity'. Below, we will employ the complex interactions that would constitute a health-promoting transport policy in a similar vein.

Public Health Systems Analysis

To understand the need for a more all-embracing approach to the formation of public health policy is merely the starting point to the development of effective interven-tions. For many years health promotion has declared that health improvement is 'everybody's business', but without clear programmatic interpretation this can sim-ply translate into 'nobody's responsibility'. Thus, amongst the oft-perplexing myriad of influences (the Foresight Report's initial systems map, for example, was so inclusive and detailed that it was illegible to the naked eye) it is necessary to isolate and prioritise. To find the necessary tools for this, public health must co-opt analytic tools more fully developed and previously more extensively employed in other fields of scientific and social scientific investigation (Joffe and Mindell 2006). By borrowing from elsewhere, it will be possible to build a loose 'toolkit' which might generically be thought of as *Public Health Systems Analysis*.

To 'de-construct' its initial systems map, with a view to isolating effective points of policy intervention, the Foresight Committee drew upon the approach of *causal loop modelling* which produced a series of individual maps which were then fused together to produce a composite atlas. This approach is illustrated in the appendices to the Committee's report (Vandenbroek et al. 2007a, 2007b). The Committee then incorporated a simplified map which clustered areas thematically and identified critical spheres of influence and the most important actors within them.

The Foresight Committee was operating at what might be thought of as the 'macro' level—identifying broad areas for meaningful intervention and the policy actors that must be 'brought to the table'. Working at the micro level requires a more detailed analysis which draws in 'ground level' participation. Yet again, we might find that practical work undertaken in developing countries (see, for example, Suba et al. 2006) might pre-figure that needed by their more developed counterparts.

Elsewhere (Thunhurst 2012) it has been suggested that there are three stages to the analysis of complex public health systems: Identifying systems components and their interactions; Identifying meaningful interventions; and Strengthening the contribution of key systems actors. Illustrations are provided of the way that systems analysis tools have been deployed within each of these areas.

Community Involvement

But before we move on to the 'mechanics' of public health systems analysis, it is worth stressing an implication of adopting a whole systems approach which attains particular significance when working at the more micro level, or when translating the implementation of macro level policy formation down to the project implementation level. This is the necessity of full community engagement. The Marmot Review (Marmot 2010, p. 157) saw this as central to the adoption of a whole systems approach:

> 'Community engagement can serve as an important lever to reduce health inequalities by influencing service provision. This often operates best in small localities and the involvement of primary care services is critical. Benefits to the community extend beyond the initial intervention and through increased participation lead to greater confidence and competence among individual citizens and can bring many positive real-life changes'.

It might be thought that this is a somewhat instrumental view of community involvement—that community engagement is necessary for successful implementation. Undoubtedly, this is true. But it is also important to engage communities from the outset. Interventions within the social and economic environment do not always engender the responses that might be predicted. For example, it might be argued that the resistance to the MMR vaccine and the preference for separate individual vaccinations that was felt to obstruct the programme to tackle the individual diseases came about because popular knowledge comes from popular conversations (viz. fears of medical establishment manipulation) rather than from a detailed reading of the epidemiological literature. Popular knowledge, warts an' all, will be disregarded at the peril of programme implementation. And, to put it more positively, popular knowledge can be a most frequent source of innovation and experimentation.

A Seat at the Policy Table

This raises a critical issue for public health policy formers. Who should sit at the policy table and where, indeed, is the policy table to be found. Addressing the second question first, it should be clear that policy tables for public health can no longer be confined to those that exist in what we conventionally think of as the health sector. To adopt the Whole Systems Approach implies gaining access to those arenas where social, economic and environmental policies are determined. The recent return, within the UK, of public health to local government, which many consider to be its natural home, makes this more feasible and more likely when local policy is being determined—albeit at a time when local government is increasingly restricted in its ability to set policy in crucial areas such as within the education sector. Centrally, where sectoral decision-making is more atomised, public health sits uneasily—with relatively minor influence within or without of the conventional health sector. In one of the boldest and far-reaching national health policies recently formulated, for the Republic of Ireland (Department of Health and Children 2001), it had been proposed to give public health a seat at the cabinet table. Change of minister at a critical juncture led to this exciting prospect being shelved.

And, in respect of who should be at the table, it should be equally clear that membership of the policy arena should be inclusive. Notwithstanding the difficulties that statutory agencies have traditionally experienced with community engagement, approaching engagement as a mutual learning process can over time provide community representatives with an effective voice (see, for example, Pickin et al. (2002) and NICHE (2008) for proposals for strengthening statutory agencies' ability to engage with lay communities).

Policy Analysis

Enlarging the orbit of public health policy determination and increasing the involvement in that determination will only add to the complexity of the processes involved in predicting the health consequences of putative health, social, economic and environmental policies. Methods of Health Impact Assessment (discussed more fully below and in Thunhurst (2007)) have been developed for just such a task. They are strong on process, providing clear guidelines for inclusive engagement. But, except in trivial situations, they will need to be underpinned by more formal methods of policy analysis. These should address not only the more quantitative impacts of candidate policies (that is their impact on measurable quantities such as life expectancy and quality of life), but also the political dimensions to policy implementation—who is likely to support it, who is likely to oppose it, what will be the major hurdles to implementation. Policy mapping (or its near-variant political mapping) has been employed to structure understanding of the policy/political arena—see, for example, Glassman et al. (1999). Thunhurst (2007) includes an illustration of how methods derived from cognitive mapping were employed to clarify the understandings of respective protagonists in the debate concerning the introduction of contentious methods of waste management in Ireland, thereby highlighting how improved information flows could help to 'rationalise' this debate.

Discussion Task
A city local authority proposes to introduce a new rapid transport system. Amongst the key objectives is improvement in the health status of communities, both within the immediate catchment of the new system and within the city more widely. Outline the range of 'actors' that should be represented at the policy table. In particular identify means by which relevant community voices may be enabled.

Planning Public Health Interventions

Planning and the Planning Spiral

Policy analysis, appropriately applied, will provide the achievement of public health objectives with focus—identifying the critical arena, or more likely arenas, of intervention and establishing broad objectives for what might be achieved within them. From broad policy formation we can move into active planning of interventions. Planning may take place at a strategic or an operational level—essentially a differentiation of specificity and generally a differentiation of planning horizon. Thus, strategic planning may take place over a five year planning period; operational planning may take place over a one year planning period. We will return to the relationship between the two further below; but necessarily strategic planning will be more closely allied to and informed by the policy formation process, whereas operational planning will be more closely allied to day-to-day management. Composition of planning teams will reflect this.

Planning is conventionally undertaken according to a *planning cycle*—though, more recently, it has become the norm to refer to a *planning spiral* emphasising the progressive nature of the turns of individual cycles. The stages of the spiral are generally termed: Situational analysis; Priority, goal and objective setting; option appraisal; programming; implementation and monitoring; and evaluation. Although portrayed sequentially (representing the extent to which the proposed intervention 'hardens up') it is always stressed that the cycle is internally recursive in nature—that is, it will generally be necessary to return to prior stages in the cycle once detailed consideration has moved on to latter stages. (Discussion of the practicalities of monitoring and evaluation, for example, can frequently lead to a need to re-visit objectives to attain greater precision).

More detailed consideration of the respective stages of the planning spiral can be found elsewhere (see, for example, Green (1992)). Illustrations can also be found (Thunhurst 2013) of how the problem structuring methods of public health systems analysis can be employed within the planning process to enrich the depth and extent of participation at the various stages of that process.

(a) The Situational Analysis

The Situational Analysis provides the broad setting for the proposed arena of intervention which will have been determined in the foregoing process of policy analysis. As we have seen, for public health interventions, arenas of intervention will fall both inside and outside of the conventional health sector. It might be natural to suspect that internal interventions will be easier to design and implement than external interventions, given the more direct access to levers of control that might be available. However, experience has demonstrated that internal interventions can prove as fraught with political difficulty as external ones, and therefore each should be approached with the same degree of rigor. This will involve the identification and collection of core information on the health sector itself (for internal interventions) and core information on collaborating sectors (for external interventions). Information emanating from political/policy analysis conducted at the policy formation stage will be carried forward into the Situational Analysis to alert those responsible for implementation of likely sources of support and resistance.

(b) Priority, Goal and Objective Setting

Overall objectives for an area of intervention will largely be carried forward from the policy analysis. This will have determined the broad contribution that can be anticipated. However, as more detailed planning progresses further definition will be needed. Most critically, at this stage, fuller consideration will be given to timescale. Objectives that were specified in general aspirational terms will be 'tied-down'. To do this, active iteration with the following stage, Option Appraisal, will be essential.

(c) Option Appraisal

It is unlikely, to being almost inconceivable, that complex public health interventions can be tackled in only one way. The adoption of a whole systems approach incorporates a much richer view of the causation of poor and good health status, with complex causal pathways, interactions and feedback loops between distinct determining factors. A systems map such as that developed for the review of strategies for tackling obesity undertaken by the Foresight

Committee (Butland et al. 2007) provides a graphic representation of alternate pathways. Option appraisal involves both the identification and the evaluation of available pathways. As well as differing timescales and resource needs, this will involve reconsideration of the degree of support and opposition highlighted by the foregoing political/policy analysis.

(d) Programming

Programming involves setting a detailed timescale for an intervention, usually represented in the form of a Gantt Chart. As complex interventions require the involvement of other parties a participative approach to programming will be required. It is a relatively easy process for a representative from another sector or from the community to 'sign up' for an intervention; it may be much more difficult for them to get their colleagues or their fellow community members to engage in active participation, as may be required. Complex interventions can be undermined by an unrealistic presumption on this score and thereby lead to frustration and a sense of antagonism that other parties are not pulling their weight.

(e) Implementation and Monitoring

If prior stages in the planning cycle have been adequately addressed this should be the easiest stage. However, complex interventions necessarily include assumptions about the engagement of other parties and about conditions prevalent in the external environment (which we will return to later). With complex interventions there will also be more internal hurdles that will arise that could not be or were not anticipated. Monitoring systems should be sufficiently sensitive to alert the prime manager or management team to the failure to meet these assumptions or the presence of such hurdles. Implementation structures should enable a relatively rapid and participatory means of response.

(f) Evaluation

We will return to the issues of evaluation below since, at it will be argued, evaluation should be seen as the driving force behind and built into the core design of complex interventions. Rather than, as is far too frequently the situation, it being seen as a post-hoc activity, something that is only addressed once the intervention has been completed. It is a common experience (certainly to the author of this chapter) that meaningful evaluation of an intervention requires the availability of data which will not have been collected during the course of the intervention unless evaluation was to the fore during the initial development of the intervention.

Rolling Planning Processes

We have noted that public health planning will take place at a number of different levels. We have employed the common terminological differentiation *strategic* and *operational*. It might be more common in public health to think of these as *programmes* and *projects*. In either case, the latter will be 'nested' within the former, in that objectives for public health projects will be drawn down from umbrella programmes or, to put that the other way, the achievement of the objectives of programmes will generally be broken down into a number of distinct projects, each with more defined objectives.

In respect of the planning and implementation of constituent projects it is essential that respective mechanisms synchronise fully with the parent programme. Monitoring of projects, for example, must feedback up to programme monitoring as adjustments might be needed at this level. (It is, for example, not uncommon to find that an external condition presumed as being met for successful project implementation requires an additional intervention to be made at programme level.)

Programmes and projects will generally have differing timescales with projects being implemented over a shorter time span. Programme implementation should be seen as a rolling process. Where practical, programmes may be adjusted to cater for issues that arise within project implementation; but, issues will inevitably be thrown up within project, and within programme, implementation that lie outside of the scope of existing programme. Review mechanisms should be built into programme implementation to ensure that the process of designing successive programmes is built into the execution of the prior programme and does not become an ab initio process that begins once the current programme is completed. Again, this highlights the importance of making evaluation a live activity undertaken throughout the course of an intervention.

Evaluating Complex Public Health Interventions

There is an implied criticism, in the call for the adoption of a whole systems approach, that public health interventions have frequently been too piecemeal in their design and execution. That is, it is presumed that individual interventions will either have an unlikely level of impact on their own or that the execution of individual interventions will incrementally lead to the achievement of higher level objectives in an unplanned and generally fortuitous way.

The need to establish the broader view, and to design shorter term interventions within the umbrella of that broader viewer has long been known to planners and managers of interventions within the field of development. Here, it is well recognised that prevailing conditions of uncertainty preclude design and implementation of highly prescriptive tightly defined projects. Flexibility and adaptability are preconditions to the successful achievement of objectives. We will, below, 'borrow' a tool that has been frequently and relatively successfully employed within the development field for a number of years, that is the logical framework. But first it is necessary to consider the appropriateness of other tools more usually adopted from proximate fields of scientific enquiry.

RCTs and the 'Gold Standard' of Evidence

The randomised control trial is frequently portrayed as providing the 'gold standard' of scientific evidence. And, where there is a simple cause–effect relationship between intervention and impact this portrayal is not an unreasonable one. The efficacy of a therapeutic intervention, or of a new drug, may be relatively easily determined by a systematic examination of outcome when assessed against an alternate or placebo intervention. Using prior knowledge to establish appropriate sample size and adopting classical statistical methods can alert the investigator to significant differences in outcome and thereby an assessment of the efficacy of the intervention.

Complex interventions, by their nature, do not exhibit simple cause–effect relationships and the point of intervention is generally well removed from the point of impact. As regards the latter characteristic, enough is already well known about the sample size that is required to assess the efficacy of a diagnostic test. The outcome of a diagnostic test is not immediate impact on the patient, as this is mediated. Outcome is dependent upon how the clinician receiving test results interprets and acts upon the results of the diagnostic test. This fuzziness in the cause–effect relationship means that sample sizes required to achieve the same level of statistical power have to be increased geometrically. Public health interventions, particularly those of a whole systems nature are so far removed from the ultimate point of impact (or points of impact) to require sample sizes of astronomical proportions to gain significant results.

And, of course whole systems interventions rarely exhibit a simple cause–effect relationship however far distanced that relationship may be. Whole systems interventions are rarely mono-causal, in that they do not consist of a single intervention, and they are frequently not mono-effect. An intervention (or a series of interventions) which aims at putting an environmental change, say, on to a health enhancing footing will require attention to issues of access, affordability, etc. as well as implementation of the specific intervention itself. And the impact of the change may be spread across a series of health conditions—improvement in mental health, reduction of heart disease, decrease in respiratory disease, etc. Any individual improvement may not be considered significant in a conventional statistical sense but the cumulative impact may be considerable.

> **Discussion Task**
> Consider the range of health outcomes (positive and negative) that might result from the introduction of a rapid transport system. Identify measures that might be employed to enhance the positive effects and to mitigate against the negative effects. Would any of these measures require additional actors to be brought to the policy table?

Health Impact Assessment

Some attempt to address the shortcomings of traditional methods of evaluation have been made in the emergence of approaches of Health Impact Assessment. The World Health Organisation (2014) provides comprehensive guidance on the purpose and methods of Health Impact Assessment. That guidance is too detailed to be summarised here. A key feature in Health Impact Assessment is a high level of community involvement and the processes of Health Impact Assessment are designed so as to ensure that involvement.

Following its wide adoption within the UK, Europe and some developing nations, a recent thorough review of the applicability of Health Impact Assessment was recently undertaken within the United States (National Research Council 2011, p. 3). It concluded that:

> 'Health impact assessment (HIA) has arisen as an especially promising way to factor health considerations into the decision-making process. It has been defined in various ways but essentially is a structured process that uses scientific data, professional expertise, and stakeholder input to identify and evaluate public-health consequences of proposals and suggests actions that could be taken to minimize adverse health impacts and optimize beneficial ones. HIA has been used throughout the world to evaluate the potential health consequences of a wide array of proposals that span many sectors and levels of government'.

The Belfast Health Cities Project (Belfast Healthy Cities 2004) issues guidelines for the development of community health profiles. These were seen as fundamental to the completion of a Community Health Impact Assessment, taking HAI to the community level.

The Logical Framework

A Logical Framework may be thought of as a *model* of an intervention; that is, it is a simplified representation. As a *simplified* representation it does not tell the full story; it will require an accompanying narrative. If the intervention is of a more strategic nature the accompanying narrative will be fuller. But, particularly when used as a checklist during intervention design it can ensure that full consideration is given to the fundamental logic behind the intervention, how the intervention is to be executed, and how it is to be monitored and evaluated. And, thereby, it will ensure that evaluation is integral to the execution of the intervention.

The Logical Framework is a four-by-four matrix.

Narrative Summary (NS)	Verifiable Indicators (OVI)	Means of Verification (MoV)	Important Assumptions
Goal:			
Purpose:			
Outputs:			
1.			
2.			
3.			
4.			
5.			
Activities:			
1.1			
1.2			
:			
:			
2.1			
2.2			
:			
:			
3.1			
3.2			
:			
:			
:			
:			

(a) The Hierarchy of Objectives

The first and the last columns provide the essential logic incorporated into intervention design. The first column (the Narrative Summary, sometimes referred to as the Hierarchy of Objectives) may be read downwards as answering a series of 'How?' questions or read up to answer a series of 'Why?' questions.

The Goal will be a simple statement of the overriding objective of the intervention. It will be pitched at a high level, and it will be an objective that the intervention is unlikely to deliver on its own. Thus, it situates the intervention into a wider context and it is there to remind us why we are undertaking the intervention.

The Purpose will be a statement of the change that we anticipate that the intervention will bring about. Conventionally, it is thought that a single intervention should have a single statement of purpose. This is a good convention to attempt to follow, as it provides clarity; but with complex interventions being implemented in a context of multiple causes and multiple effects it may not always be possible to be that focussed.

The Outputs, which again for clarity should not be too numerous (six is often taken as an upper limit), can be thought of as the intervention's *deliverables*. That is, these are the objectives that the intervention is designed to deliver as a means of bringing about the change specified in the preceding Purpose level objective.

The Activities, a number of which will be attached to each specified output, will list all of those things that will need to happen to ensure that the respective output is delivered. As the intervention moves from the more strategic to the more operational level these will begin to take the form of inputs—specific resource needs.

Thus, the underlying logic of the intervention is that if the activities are undertaken then the outputs will be delivered, if the outputs are delivered then the purpose will be achieved, if the purpose is achieved then the goal will be attained (or at least the intervention's contribution to the goal will be attained). However, complex interventions are implemented in complex environments. It will always be necessary when focussing on a specific intervention to make certain assumptions about the stability of that environment or of changes in that environment which might reasonably be anticipated and which are necessary for the intervention to succeed at the respective levels.

The fourth column lists any key assumptions that are being made in the successful progression from one level in the hierarchy of objectives to the next. Thus, it would be more complete to say that that if the activities are undertaken and the assumptions made at that level are correct *then* the outputs will be delivered, if the outputs are delivered and the assumptions made at that level are correct *then* the purpose will be achieved, if the purpose is achieved and the assumptions made at that level are correct *then* the (contribution to the) goal will be attained. At the goal level we will identify the parallel interventions or conditions for the achievement of the goal.

A thorough process of intervention design will involve a risk assessment—essentially an appraisal of the likelihood that stipulated assumptions will be met. Where there is high risk that an important assumption will not be met intervention design should be modified accordingly.

(b) Monitoring and Evaluation

This leaves the two inner columns—the Verifiable Indicators and the Means of Verification. For each objective, at every level, it will be necessary to specify how attainment of that objective will be verified. This may be in the form of a quantitative indicator, or a set of quantitative indicators, or it may be in the form of a qualitative indicator or indicators, or some combination of both. The former are often preferred, as they are generally simpler to calibrate and easier to analyse. These indicators are listed in the Verifiable Indicators (OVI) column. (The 'O' standing for the generally redundant 'Observable' which had been part of earlier terminology.)

For each indicator it is necessary to specify the means by which the calibrating data will be collected—the Means of Verification. This column is necessary, since in data-poor contexts, calibration of the indicator may be reliant upon sources which are either non-existing, unreliable or extremely costly to establish. [It is by no means unusual, at the early drafting stage, for members of a design team to specify an indicator which would be more costly to collect - requiring whole population survey, say—than would the implementation of the intervention itself].

Project monitoring is the process of ensuring that project activities are undertaken as specified and that project outputs are delivered. Thus the project monitoring system may be thought of as being contained within the area of the logical framework shaded below:

Narrative Summary (NS)	Verifiable Indicators (OVI)	Means of Verification (MoV)	Important Assumptions
Goal:			
Purpose:			
Outputs:			
1.			
2.			
3.			
4.			
5.			
Activities:			
1.1			
1.2			
:			
:			
2.1			
2.2			
:			
:			
3.1			
3.2			
:			
:			
:			
:			

Project evaluation is the process of ensuring that the project outputs are delivered and that the change specified in the project purpose is attained. Thus the project evaluation system may be thought of as being contained within the area of the logical framework shaded below:

Narrative Summary (NS)	Verifiable Indicators (OVI)	Means of Verification (MoV)	Important Assumptions
Goal:			
Purpose:			
Outputs:			
1.			
2.			
3.			
4.			
5.			
Activities:			
1.1			
1.2			
:			
:			
2.1			
2.2			
:			
:			
3.1			
3.2			
:			
:			
:			
:			

(c) The Accompanying Narrative

The conciseness of the summary provided by the logical framework necessarily means that not all key issues can be addressed within it. Some explanation will be necessary of the logic implicit within the hierarchy of objectives and the Important Assumptions. As mentioned, a risk assessment will appraise the likelihood attached to the respective assumptions. As many of these will involve the actions of external partners, this may entail what is called a *stakeholder analysis*. And the achievement of the stated objectives will rarely be trivial; some statement of processes will be needed. It is most likely that an intervention formulated at the more strategic level will require a much fuller narrative summary as the degree of interdependence with external factors will be greater.

(d) An Hierarchy of Logical Frameworks

Interventions at the strategic level will generally be implemented through a series of interventions at the operational level. (A programme will comprise or contain a number of projects). This implicitly means an additional level to the hierarchy of objectives. However, this is attained by 'nesting' a set of lower level logical frameworks into the higher level logical framework. In essence, the outputs of the programme logical framework become the purposes for the respective project logical frameworks (and the activities of the programme become the outputs of the projects).

For complex projects, an element of further decomposition may also be needed. Lower level logical frameworks may be developed for each of the outputs (which now themselves become individual purposes). In this manner, it is very clear to those project participants whose contribution may be at a very detailed level how their contribution fits in (indeed, is critical) to the attainment of the project and programme goals at the higher level.

Discussion Task

Consider a city known to you. Draw up a broad (outline) logical framework for the introduction of a rapid transport systems. Draw up a more detailed logical framework for an output level objective within that logical framework (to become a purpose level objective in the more detailed logical framework) which is 'To ensure that the potential health advantages of the rapid transport system are maximised and that any potential negative health impacts are minimised'.

Information Needs

Superficially it may be thought that careful attention to the development of a logical framework will enable immediate and simple definition of data needs and data sources. And this will largely be the case. However, there are two important areas where capturing the necessary data may not be a trivial matter.

The Community-Based Health Information Network

The importance of full community engagement to the implementation of complex public health interventions has been stressed. The whole systems approach requires change at all levels. The most critical will often be those changes designed together with and implemented at the community level. This is where data may be most sparse. As well as quite detailed geographically disaggregated 'hard' data on prevailing health conditions, 'softer' data on beliefs, understandings, attitudes and behaviours will be needed—both to ensure realistic design of interventions and because these will often be the focus of desired change.

Such detailed local information is rarely available and whole population data collection will rarely be feasible. This will be particularly the case when the key participant group in an intervention may be a minority group which generally exhibit high levels of mobility and/or a reluctance to provide information to 'official' data collectors.

Such data scarcity is not unfamiliar to project and programme implementers from developing countries. In such contexts it is the norm to employ methods of *rapid appraisal*. At the heart of rapid appraisal methods is the use of *key informants*. These are either members of a community or key workers within the community knowledgeable of the health situation of, and the health beliefs and behaviours prevalent within, that community. As part of a recent investigation to build a health profile of one 'hard-to-reach' area within Coventry it was proposed to build a community-based health information network composed of a comprehensive set of key informants from within that community (Fig. 1).

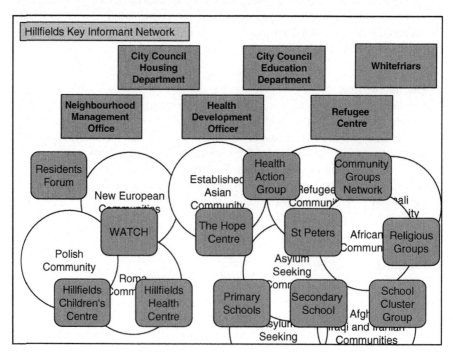

Fig. 1 A community-based health information network (from Thunhurst 2009)

Inter-sectoral Information

A whole systems approach requires not only the active participation of other sectors but a regular flow of information. This will be needed both for the calibration of key Verifiable Indicators and to monitor whether key assumptions relating to those sectors have been met. The recent tendency towards the fragmentation of local services and the accompanying trend to declare important areas of data 'commercial in confidence' have made inter-sectoral information gathering considerably more problematic. (For example, to establish pattern of public transport usage within a British city would now involve the cooperation of a myriad of local operatives.) Public health has a keen interest in the early stages of the 'contracting out' process, ensuring the regular flow of key data and incorporation of public health objectives into relevant performance standards.

Discussion Task
Drawing upon the logical framework developed in earlier activity and upon any other pertinent considerations, identify the data needed for effective monitoring and evaluation of the health impact of the introduction of the rapid transport system. What will be the sources of these data? Will any new structures or processes be needed to ensure the generation of these data?

Conclusion

This chapter has explored the health intelligence needs of a critical but oft-neglected sphere of public health practice—the formulation of policy, the planning of public health interventions and the monitoring and evaluation of those interventions. Public health practitioners are frequently called upon to respond to immediate crises; but their most effective long term impact on health status is achieved when they implement or combine with others to implement policies aimed at achieving more fundamental change in the conditions which generate good or bad health outcomes. Given the protracted timescale over which such intervention may be implemented and the multitude of agencies that may be involved in the implementation, it is all too easy to ignore intelligence needs until the implementation is complete. Retrospectively, we seek to answer the questions 'well, how did it go?' and 'what have we achieved?'; at this point we find that the requisite health intelligence is lacking and the questions can not be answered definitively. In this chapter we have advocated the use of a logical framework approach which, if thoroughly and appropriately applied, will ensure that intelligence needs are to the forefront throughout the process of intervention design and thereby also throughout the intervention itself.

Recommended Reading

The Whole Systems Approach to Public Health

Fuller elaboration of the pre-history to the emergence of the Whole Systems Approach is given in recent articles by the current author (Thunhurst 2012, 2013). Compelling evidence of the need for such an approach is provided by the respective reports of the Commission on the Social Determinants of Health (WHO 2008) and the Marmot Review (Marmot 2010)

Public Health Systems Analysis

Public Health Systems Analysis draws heavily upon the *Problem Structuring Methods* developed as a distinct field within operational research. The most comprehensive guide to these is the textbook edited by Rosenhead and Mingers (2001)

Health Impact Assessment

Numerous examples of the use of Health Impact Assessment have now been published. The most accessible guide to the conduct of Health Impact Assessment is to be found on the WHO website (WHO 2014)

The Logical Framework

Guidance on the construction of a logical framework can be found in the literature on project management (see, for example, Jackson (1997)). For consideration of their use in health policy and planning, see Nancholas (1998).

References

Barton, H., & Grant, M. (2006). A health map for the local human habitat. *The Journal for the Royal Society for the Promotion of Health, 126*(6), 252–253. doi:10.1177/1466424006070466.
Belfast Healthy Cities. (2004). *Developing a community profile: Guidelines*. Belfast, Ireland: Belfast Healthy Cities.
Butland, B., Jebb, S., Kopelman, P., McPherson, K., Thomas, S., Mardell, J. et al. (2007). *Foresight. Tackling obesities: Future choices—Project Report*. Government Office for Science: London, England. Accessed September 23, 2015, from https://www.gov.uk/government/uploads/system/uploads/attachment_data/file/287937/07-1184x-tackling-obesities-future-choices-report.pdf

Dahlgren, G., & Whitehead, M. (1991). *Policies and strategies to promote social equity in health.* Stockholm: Institute of Futures Studies.

Department of Health and Children. (2001). *Quality and fairness—A health system for you.* Dublin: The Stationery Office.

Friel, S., Hattersley, L., & Townsend, R. (2015). Trade policy and public health. *Annual Review of Public Health, 36*, 325–344.

Glassman, A., Reich, M. R., Laserson, K., & Rojas, F. (1999). Political analysis of health reform in the Dominican Republic. *Health Policy and Planning, 14*(2), 115–126.

Green, A. (1992). *An introduction to health planning in developing countries.* Oxford, England: Oxford University Press.

Jackson, B. (1997). *Designing projects and project evaluations using the logical framework approach. IUCN monitoring and evaluation initiative.* Retrieved January 2, 2015, from http://cmsdata.iucn.org/downloads/logframepaper3.pdf.

Joffe, M., & Mindell, J. (2006). Complex causal process diagrams for analysing the health impacts of policy interventions. *American Journal of Public Health, 96*, 473–479.

Kuh, D., & Ben-Shlomo, Y. (2004). *A life course approach to chronic disease epidemiology.* Oxford, England: Oxford University Press.

Marmot, M. (2010). *The Marmot review: Fair society, healthy lives.* London: UCL. Retrieved January 2, 2015, from https://www.instituteofhealthequity.org/projects/fair-society-healthy-lives-the-marmot-review.

Nancholas, S. (1998). How to do (or not to do) … a logical framework. *Health Policy and Planning, 13*(2), 189–193.

National Institute for Health and Clinical Excellence. (2008). *Community Engagement to improve health* (NICE public health guidance, Vol. 9). London: NICE.

National Institute for Health and Clinical Excellence. (2010). *Preventing obesity using a 'whole-system' approach at local and community level - Public Health Guidance, Draft Scope.* London: NICE.

National Research Council. (2011). *Committee on Health Impact Assessment; National Research Council.* Washington DC: The National Academies Press. Improving Health in the United States: The Role of Health Impact Assessment, Retrieved December 31, 2015, from http://www.nap.edu/catalog.php?record_id=13229.

Pickin, C., Popay, J., Staely, K., Bruce, N., Jones, C., & Gowman, N. (2002). Developing a model to enhance the capacity of statutory organisations to engage with lay communities. *Journal of Health Services Research and Policy, 7*(1), 34–42.

Rosenhead, J., & Mingers, J. (2001). *Rational Analysis for a Problematic World* (2nd ed.). Chichester, England: John Wiley.

Suba, E., Murphy, S., Donnelly, A., Furia, L., Huynh, M., & Raab, S. (2006). Systems analysis of real-world obstacles to successful cervical cancer prevention in developing countries. *American Journal of Public Health, 96*, 480–487.

Thunhurst, C. (2007). Refocusing Upstream: Operational Research for population health. *Journal of the Operational Research Society, 58*, 186–194.

Thunhurst, C. (2009). Measuring the health of urban populations: What progress have we made? *Public Health, 123*(1), e40–e44. doi:10.1016/j.puhe.2008.10.016.

Thunhurst, C. (2012). Public health systems analysis—The transfer of learning between developed and developing countries. *Health Care Management Science, 15*(3), 283–291. doi:10.1007/s10729-012-9192-0.

Thunhurst, C. (2013). Public health systems analysis—Where the River Kabul meets the River Indus. *Globalization and Health, 9*, 39.

Vandenbroek, P., Goossens, J., & Clemens, M. (2007a). *Tackling obesities: Future choices—Building the obesity system map.* London: Government Office for Science. Retrieved September 23, 2015, from https://www.gov.uk/government/uploads/system/uploads/attachment_data/file/295154/07-1179-obesity-building-system-map.pdf.

Vandenbroek, P., Goossens, J., & Clemens, M. (2007b). *Tackling obesities: Future choices—Obesity system atlas*. London: Government Office for Science. Retrieved September 23, 2015, from https://www.gov.uk/government/uploads/system/uploads/attachment_data/file/295153/07-1177-obesity-system-atlas.pdf.

World Health Organisation. (2008). *Closing the gap in a generation*. Geneva, Switzerland: WHO Commission on Social Determinants of Health. Retrieved September 23, 2015, from http://www.who.int/social_determinants/thecommission/finalreport/en/.

World Health Organisation. (2014). Health impact assessment. Retrieved September 23, 2015, from http://www.who.int/hia/en/

Health Needs Assessment

Patrick Tobi

Abstract Health needs assessment (HNA) is one of the approaches used to provide intelligence and inform decision-making on the planning and deploying of resources to address the health priorities of local populations. Need is an important concept in public health but is also a multifaceted one that represents different things to different people. From a public health perspective, need is seen as the 'ability to benefit', which means that there must be effective interventions available to meet the need. In present-day public health practice, assessing the health needs of local populations typically involves considering not just their physical and mental health and well-being, but the wider determinants or social factors, such as housing, employment and education that influence their health. This chapter describes the historic development of health needs assessment and its use in contemporary public health practice. The different ways in which need is perceived and their implications for the health service are discussed. A step-by-step guide through the HNA process is outlined and comparisons are made with other overlapping approaches to assessment. The practical challenges of carrying out HNAs are highlighted and case studies are used to illustrate real life experiences.

By the end of this chapter, you should be able to:

- Discuss the concepts of need, want and demand.
- Describe what is meant by a health needs assessment (HNA) and the different approaches that currently influence thinking and practice underpinning HNA.
- Identify the key steps and practical challenges involved in conducting a HNA.
- Compare HNA with other overlapping assessment approaches.
- Understand, through case studies, how HNA is applied in practice.

P. Tobi (✉)
Institute for Health and Human Development, University of East London,
Water Lane, Stratford, UK
e-mail: p.tobi@uel.ac.uk

© Springer International Publishing Switzerland 2016   169
K. Regmi, I. Gee (eds.), *Public Health Intelligence*,
DOI 10.1007/978-3-319-28326-5_9

Introduction

Health needs assessment (HNA) is one of a number of approaches that are commonly used by practitioners and service commissioners across all sectors to inform decision-making. The term was coined in the early 1990s; a period dominated by the 'medical model' of health which had a strong emphasis on disease and illness. Notwithstanding advocacy by bodies such as the World Health Organisation (WHO) who argued for a definition of health based on well-being, and not merely the absence of disease or infirmity, public health at the time was, perhaps not surprisingly, oriented towards disease and healthcare. HNAs were typically conducted around disease conditions or services, for example, diabetes, cancer, heart disease and child health services. The terms HNA and healthcare needs assessment (HCNA) also tended to be used interchangeably. From the late 1990s, the emphasis of HNA shifted as the well-being perspective of health gained ground and public health and Government health policy changed in line with increasing recognition of the influence of the wider social and environmental factors that impact on health, such as education, employment, housing and deprivation.

What Is Health Needs Assessment?

HNA is a systematic method for reviewing the health issues facing a population, leading to agreed priorities and resource allocation that will improve health and reduce inequalities (Cavanagh and Chadwick 2005, p. 6). It is a practical and structured process of planning and deploying resources to identify and address the health priorities of local populations and create health gain. Another useful definition comes from Wright (2001) who described HNA as a systematic public health process for identifying the unmet health and healthcare needs of a population, making changes to meet those needs and creating health gain. In recent times, the emphasis of HNA has moved towards the objective of achieving equity, i.e. fair user access to services and fair resource allocation (Powell 2006).

The concept and practice of HNA developed during the 1990s (Stevens and Rafferty 1994, 1997) and it is now a well-established process for determining a population's health priorities and informing commissioning and service planning. Contemporary descriptions of HNA embrace populations rather than diseases or healthcare services as the starting point of assessment. The population may be defined by geography, social characteristics, health condition or any other relevant criteria. The role of multi-sector partnerships and engagement with the target community or population in the process is also highlighted. While HNA may be defined in slightly different ways, some common themes or concepts are evident in the definitions:

- *Systematic*—an organised approach, structured process or method behind the HNA.

- *Population*—people or communities are the starting point of the process.
- *Partnership*—involving other stakeholders, including target communities, in the process.
- *Identification of need*—gathering and assessing information about health issues.
- *Prioritisation and resourcing*—agreeing priorities and allocating resources.
- *Action*—making changes (deploying resources and interventions) to address the need.

Some other forms of assessment are also used to help improve health and reduce health inequalities including Health Impact Assessment (HIA), Integrated Impact Assessment (IIA) and Health Equity Audit (HEA). Quigley et al. (2005) noted that while they have overlapping areas of interest and so share some similarities with HNA, they also differ in certain aspects. Table 1 summarises the main features of some of the more common assessment approaches.

> **Discussion Task**
> What do we mean by Health Needs Assessment?
>
> **Comments**: Assessing the health and healthcare needs of the local population is a fundamental part of many public health activities (from Powell 2006, p. 146). One way this can be done is through a health needs assessment. Other overlapping approaches include equity audit, impact assessment, policy/planning review, target setting, resource allocation, and evaluation of current and potential services.

The Concept of Need

Need is a complex concept and can mean different things to different people. It is used by both health and non-health professionals in different and varying contexts. Bradshaw's (1972) classic taxonomy of needs identified four ways in which need is perceived.

- **Normative need**—refers to what expert opinion defines as need, e.g. the need for medical treatment. It is based on professional judgment. Normative needs are not absolute and there may be different standards laid down by different experts.
- **Felt need**—what people say they want or feel they need. Felt needs are influenced by people's perceptions, knowledge and expectations of services.
- **Expressed need**—communication of felt need. This is equivalent to the demand for services and can be conveyed vocally, through people's help-seeking behaviour or the way they use services. Demand is influenced by a range of factors including illness behaviour, knowledge of services and availability (supply) of services. Not all felt need is expressed as demand.
- **Comparative need**—based on judgments by professionals as to the relative needs of different groups. It is derived from examining the services provided to

Table 1 Comparison of common features and tasks of different assessment approaches (*Source*: Quigley et al. 2005)

	Health needs assessment	Health impact assessment	Integrated impact assessment	Health equity audit
Starting point	Population	Proposal	Proposal	Services and resources
Primary output	Informs decisions about strategies, service priorities, commissioning and local delivery plans, and informs future HIAs and IIAs	Recommends how to maximise benefits and minimise negatives of a proposal to inform decision making and improve joined-up working	Recommends how to maximise benefits and minimise negatives of a proposal to inform decision making and improve joined-up working	Agreed and acted upon interventions that equitably distribute services and resources
Aims to take account of inequalities	Describes health needs and health assets of different groups in local population. Helps improve health and reduce health inequalities	Compares impact of proposals on most vulnerable groups in the population. Helps improve health and reduce health inequalities	Compares impact of proposals on most vulnerable groups in the population. Helps improve health and reduce health inequalities	Compares health needs and outcomes in the local population with use and access to services and resources. Helps improve health and reduce inequalities
Involvement of stakeholders	Always	Always	Always	Always
Involvement of community	Always	Ideally (dependent on resources)	Ideally (dependent on resources)	No
Involvement from many sectors	Sometimes	Usually	Always	Always
Based on determinants of health	Usually	Ideally	Always	Usually
Best available evidence used	Always	Always	Always	Always
Uses data from other approaches; informs other approaches	Always	Always	Always	Always

a population in one area and using this information as the basis to determine the sort of services required in another area with a similar population.

An understanding of the different dimensions of need is important to increase the chance of building a comprehensive picture of community problems. Bradshaw suggested that the four dimensions overlapped and that somewhere in the overlap *real* need could be found. He proposed that policy makers allocating scarce resources should focus on real need rather than (just) normative need, felt need, demand or comparative need (Bradshaw 1994).

From a healthcare standpoint, the notion of need is somewhat different. Health need is seen as the 'capacity to benefit'. It depends on the potential of health services to prevent or treat health problems, or mitigate their consequences. There will be no benefit to be had if there are no effective interventions or resources available. In essence, need is acknowledged to exist when there is an effective intervention available, or the potential for health gain. Behind this perspective is an important health economic principle—the recognition that the resources available to meet needs are limited. So only those health issues for which something can be done are taken into consideration.

In reality however, it is rare to find a situation where no intervention exists and there will in most cases be some option available. However, it is also important to remember that there will be no benefit from an intervention that is not effective. In the 1990s, there was an increased focus on identifying and prioritising health interventions that were supported by research evidence of effectiveness. It is for this reason that HNAs will typically include a reference to the evidence of effectiveness.

Need is distinct from demand and supply. Stevens et al. (2004) viewed need as what people might benefit from, demand as what people would be willing to pay for in a market or might wish to use in a system of free healthcare, and supply as what was actually provided, this often being determined by political priorities and available resources. At the same time, need, demand and supply also overlap to various degrees. Figure 1 shows the following configurations of overlap:

An understanding of the relationship between the three areas might further assist in guiding commissioning decisions on investment and disinvestment of resources so that services are able to better direct supply to where it is most needed. This is illustrated in Fig. 2.

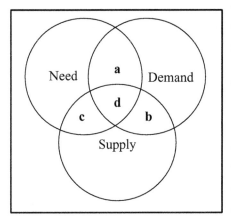

a. **Unmet need:** need is felt and expressed as demand but not identified as a normative need by the health service.

b. **Inappropriate supply:** need is not felt, but nevertheless is expressed as demand and identified as a normative need.

c. **Supplied Need:** need is felt and not expressed as demand, but is recognized by the service as a normative need.

d. **Normative Need:** need is felt, expressed as demand and supplied as a normative need.

Fig. 1 Need, demand and supply.

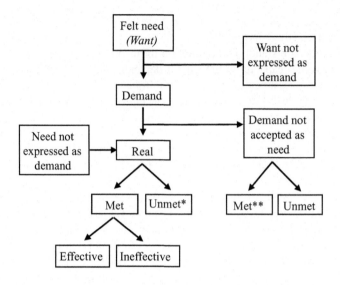

* Opportunity for health gain
** Opportunity for disinvestment with no health loss

Fig. 2 Need, demand, supply and health gain potential (*Source*: Rogers and Fox 2005)

Discussion Task
What are the differences between need, demand and supply?

Comments: In the context of healthcare needs assessment, Stevens and Raftery (1994) consider need, demand and supply in an approach that includes important health economic principles. In their view: (a) need—is the population's ability to benefit from health and social care interventions, (b) demand—is what people would be willing to pay for in a market or might wish to use in a system of free healthcare, whereas (c) supply—is provided and is often determined by political and political priorities and available resources.

Approaches to HNA

There are different ways of carrying out health needs assessments. They all share the same objective of utilising available resources in the most effective way to maximise population health benefit. Three main approaches to HNA have been described: epidemiological, comparative and corporate. The approaches are summarised in Fig. 3.

1. *Epidemiological*. This refers to the traditional public health approach of describing need in relation to specific health conditions using estimates of the incidence,

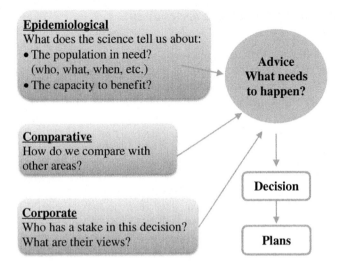

Fig. 3 HNA approaches (*Source*: Elkheir and Lambert cited in Rida Elkheir 2007, p.82)

prevalence and other indicators of health impact derived from studies carried out locally or elsewhere (Williams and Wright 1998). This approach considers the epidemiology of the condition, current service provision, and the effectiveness and cost-effectiveness of interventions and services. It, however, does not capture the perspectives of service users or the local community.

2. *Comparative*. In this approach, levels of service provision between different populations are compared. It should be borne in mind that local population characteristics (demography, mortality, morbidity, etc.) and other factors may also account for any observed differences in service use between the populations (Stevens et al. 2004).

3. *Corporate*. This approach involves the systematic collection of the knowledge and views of local stakeholders—health professionals, service-users, the public, policymakers and politicians—on healthcare services and needs (Stevens and Gillam 1998). It has been encouraged by government policy reforms that emphasised more 'local voices', patient and public involvement, partnership and collaboration. Although the corporate approach blurs the difference between need and demand, and between scientific inquiry and vested interest, elements of the approach (i.e. community engagement and user involvement) are sensitive to local circumstances and play an important role in informing local policy (Stevens et al. 2004).

Discussion Task
What are the strengths and weaknesses of the different approaches to HNA?

Conducting a Health Needs Assessment

In practice, HNAs are not carried out solely using one approach, but often incorporate elements of all three. The approach chosen may be modified to suit the local context. It is also influenced by the time and resources available to conduct the HNA. Regardless of which approach is taken, Hooper and Longworth (2002, p. 9) suggested three core principles that should underpin the entire HNA process if it is to succeed in engaging those services that are most influential in achieving health gain in those with the most to gain:

1. Improvement of health and inequalities by making changes that improve the most significant factors affecting health, then targeting the population groups with the most to gain, and those services that can make the most difference to their needs.
2. Integration of this improvement in health into the planning processes used by those services, so that the identified changes are implemented in their plans.
3. Involvement of people who know about the health issues in a community, people who care about those issues and people who can make changes happen.

There are different activities involved in carrying out a HNA, for instance health profiling, undertaking a rapid appraisal exercise, and community engagement. All the activities can be grouped under five main steps (Cavanagh and Chadwick 2005; Hooper and Longworth 2002). These are detailed in Table 2 as a series of questions or statements drawing attention to the type of activity required. For the propose of clarity the steps are described as linear, but in practice, the process will be iterative and involve moving back and forth across steps to cross-check information and make revisions where necessary.

The starting point of the process is the population and they should be clearly identified from the beginning as part of the preparation stage. The population may be defined in different ways, e.g. by geographic location, by social characteristics (age, sex, ethnicity, marital status, religion, education, occupation), by social circumstances (deprivation, homelessness, poverty), by health condition or any other appropriate attribute. It is important to ensure that all relevant partners/stakeholders are involved from the onset, particularly senior decision makers who have the power or influence to make change happen. Stakeholders in a HNA will typically cut across the statutory (local authority, local national health service), voluntary and other sectors. Consideration should be given to the resources (time, staff, skills, data availability, money, etc.) that will be needed. Threats to completing the HNA should also be identified and a risk register developed.

In developing a profile of the population, data on social, demographic and health indicators such as population size, age/sex distribution, life expectancy, mortality and morbidity rates, lifestyle measures (smoking, drinking, exercise, diet, etc.) will be gathered. The profile will include data on the most important health issues affecting the population as determined by the severity and size of the issue. It is important to also collect information on the wider or social determinants of health (housing, employment, crime, deprivation, etc.). Dahlgren and Whitehead's model (Fig. 4) is a widely

Table 2 Steps in HNA

Step 1:	*Getting started (agree aims, objectives and framework)*
(a)	Who is the population to be assessed?
(b)	What is the purpose of the assessment?
(c)	What are the boundaries of the assessment?
(d)	Who should be involved in the process?
(e)	What resources are required?
(f)	What are the risks?
Step 2:	*Identifying the health priorities for the population*
(a)	Population profiling—what are the important aspects of health functioning?
(b)	What data/information is currently available?
(c)	Perceptions of needs
(d)	Identifying and assessing health conditions and determinant factors
Step 3:	*Assessing the specific health priorities for action*
(a)	Review step 1 for this priority
(b)	What are the health conditions and determinant/factors with the most significant size and severity impact and changeability?
(c)	What are the effective and acceptable actions (in terms of impact and changeability)?
(d)	What are the resource implications?
Step 4:	*Action planning for change*
(a)	What are the aims, objectives, indicators and targets of the intervention?
(b)	Action planning—what actions need to be designed?
(c)	What should be the monitoring and evaluation strategy?
(d)	What is the risk-management strategy?
Step 5:	*Evaluation (moving on/review—learning from the intervention, measuring impact)*
(a)	Who is the evaluation for?
(b)	What are the processes and outcomes of the evaluation?

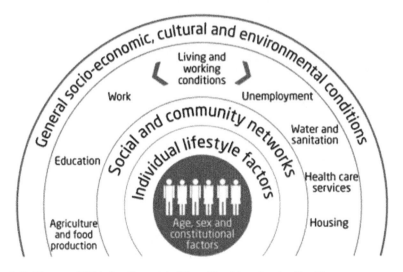

Fig. 4 Dahlgren and Whitehead's model of the wider determinants of health

used framework that helps identify the range of social determinants that influence health and upon which interventions could be based. It highlights the relationship between individual lifestyle 'choices', social networks, working and living conditions and economic, political and environmental factors (Dahlgren and Whitehead 1991).

The method of data collection will depend on the nature of data required, but almost always involves a mix of quantitative and qualitative methods. Most often, data gathering will begin with desk research to bring together and review existing data. This will be in various forms such as health profiles, surveys, service use registers, and project monitoring and evaluation reports. Primary data may need to be collected where no information exists, or the information is out of date. Qualitative methods (interviews, focus groups, observation, etc.) should be used to generate information where the issues of interest are best addressed by such methods.

After the profiling is completed, the next task is to identify the priority issues. Hooper and Longworth (2002) suggested that they could be ranked on the criteria of *impact* (severity and size of the problem) and *changeability* (potential for issue to be addressed by available and effective interventions and resources). Issues may also be prioritised as a result of community or political pressure, or because of difficulties within an existing service (Rogers and Fox 2005). The best interventions to address the issues identified in the population profiling also need to be determined. Again, this is done using an agreed set of criteria. These will include factors such as evidence of effectiveness, or examples of innovative or good practice where evidence base has not yet been established. The resources required to deliver the intervention will also be assessed.

A HNA should always lead to positive action. Accordingly, action planning, implementation, and dissemination strategies are an essential part of the process (Cavanagh and Chadwick 2005). Action planning will include agreeing aims, objectives, indicators and targets, and what should happen to implement the changes. The full cycle of HNA includes reviewing or evaluating the outcomes. The evaluation should be designed to understand the effect of the changes, both in terms of *outcome* (change in the health of the population, particularly those most at risk from the agreed health need priorities) and *process* (the service changes that were effected).

Two case studies are presented below to illustrate real life examples of conducting HNA. The population settings are a housing estate in a deprived area and a prison population. The case studies show the activities carried out in relation to the five main steps of the HNA process.

Case study 1: Health needs assessment of primary care in an isolated housing estate	
Step 1: getting started	
What population and why?	The population of a deprived housing estate in Torfaen, a county borough in Wales. Local GPs intended to withdraw from the health centre on the estate, reducing access.
Aims	• Assess the population need for primary healthcare
	• Identify ways of meeting that need

Case study 1: Health needs assessment of primary care in an isolated housing estate	
Objectives	• Describe the population and its main health needs
	• Consult community and stakeholders about determinants of health and priorities
	• Identify suitable models of care and levels of service
	• Consult the local community regarding models of care
	• Develop a business case for the establishment of the preferred service model
	• Identify evaluation criteria for the service adopted
Who was in the project team?	A specialist registrar in public health, two community development officers (LHB and voluntary sector), an LHB planning officer, a health visitor and a midwife
Which stakeholders were involved?	Torfaen County Borough Council, Torfaen Voluntary Alliance, local schools, health visitors, district nurses and midwives, primary care teams, councillors, Action Team for Jobs, Surestart, Drug and alcohol team, community pharmacist, Church of England vicar, local residents
Step 2: Identifying health priorities	
What data were available on the health of the population?	*Office of National Statistics (ONS)*: demography, mortality, morbidity, households with dependent children, socio-economic status, transport, housing
	Torfaen Health & Environment Survey: household income, problems with housing, satisfaction with environment, lifestyle, morbidity *PEDW*: hospital admissions. *Torfaen LHB*: GP registrations. *WAG*: primary care staffing
How was information gathered about the population and provider perceptions of needs?	Semi-structured interviews with stakeholders and primary care teams, and public meeting
Any barriers encountered?	Very little data available about primary care use by the population
How were these overcome?	The LHB paid practices to extract data on the relevant postcodes. The quality and usefulness of this data was poor
What were the key issues for the population?	Access to services, poverty, antisocial behaviour, lack of available mental health services
What priorities were chosen?	Provision of accessible services within the estate
Step 3: assessing a priority for action	
What interventions were considered most effective and acceptable?	Provision of open-access Nurse Practitioner service, available to all residents, and including mental health input
What changes were required?	Employment of Nurse Practitioner (by LHB) and mental health nurse (via service level agreement with Gwent Trust)
How were resource needs met?	Met by LHB out of existing funding
Step 4: action planning	
Summary of the action planning process	The LHB and CHC jointly produced a long-list of options, which was circulated for comments. A shortlist of options was taken to public consultation. The LHB board approved the establishment of the Nurse Practitioner service, and the subsequent business plan

Case study 1: Health needs assessment of primary care in an isolated housing estate	
Step 5: Moving on/review	
What did the project achieve?	Access to primary care services ensured. The needs assessment process and outcome gained the support of an initially suspicious community
How did it contribute to reducing inequalities?	Provided easy access to primary care for a deprived community, over and above that provided by their GPs
What needs to happen next?	Evaluation of the Nurse Practitioner service
What main message from this HNA will you take forward to the next?	The process of HNA is beneficial as long as it leads to change. The population was sceptical that the needs assessment was anything other than a PR tool. If no change had resulted, this impression would have been confirmed and the population would have been disinclined to participate in any future work

Source: Rogers and Fox (2005)

Case study 2: Health needs assessment within Durham cluster of prisons	
Step 1: Getting started	
What population, where located and why chosen?	Three Durham prisons (HMP Frankland, HMP Durham and HMP Low Newton)
	Prison population reveals strong evidence of health inequalities and social exclusion
	Prisoners are largely from lower socio-economic groups
	Prisoners tend to have poorer physical and mental and social health than the general population
What were the aims and objectives?	To build a picture of the current health services; assess inmates' unmet needs; plan, negotiate and make necessary changes within Durham cluster of prisons. To identify ways prisoners could have access to the same quality and range of health services as the general public
	Designing and developing a framework to gather evidence-based information using available data and organising interviews and focus groups
Who was included in the project team? Who was included in the stakeholder group?	Involving various stakeholders such as prisoners, prison health service managers, prison governors, prison officers, board of governors, PCT chief executive, PCT lay member and NHS trust. Building on information from HNA to set up a plan of action designed to meet the needs and develop HIMP for prisoners
Step 2: Identifying health priorities	
How was a profile of the population developed?	Each prison had specific type of population: female, male, sentenced, remand. The prison profile of the population was developed according to age band and what category population they belonged to, and was compared with that of the whole of County Durham
What data were available on the health of the population? How was Information gathered about the population's and service providers' perceptions of needs?	Various information sources (epidemiological, corporate and comparative data) were used to collect health-related data for quality and accuracy control. To facilitate collection of appropriate information, chart templates were designed and sent to prison healthcare staff. Very limited health data information is collected in each prison, so health information data from inmates' medical records and prescribed medication for a 3-month period was used

Case study 2: Health needs assessment within Durham cluster of prisons	
Any barriers encountered?	Lack of data information and IT system within prisons, incomplete information, lack of easy access to enter prisons, uncertainty of some staff regarding the change within the prison service
How were these overcome?	The necessary data were obtained by designing a template to collect specific data within a defined period of time. Staff were given the necessary information and appropriate explanation
What were the key issues for the population?	The average daily population in prisons has increased. 51 % of male prisoners in Durham prisons are on remand and 49 % sentenced, the majority of male inmates are aged between 20 and 39, while the average age of female inmates is 25–44 years
What priorities were chosen and why, in terms of impact and changeability?	Workforce development, staff training, improved access to primary care services, health promotion and clinical governance; issues connected to substance misuse, mental health, management of suicide and self-harm; development of the computer system
What evidence informed your decision?	Baseline information, the high number of prisoners with mental health disorders, or who are drug misusers, or both. Weakness in healthcare management, skill mix duties, lack of health risk management, inappropriate use of staff skills
Step 3: Assessing a priority for action	
What interventions were considered most effective and acceptable?	Appointment of a clinical nurse manager to ensure clinical and managerial staff uses their skills appropriately. There was evidence that strong leadership would improve clinical health services
	Training for workforce development, improvement in appointment systems within primary care
	Clinical and audit performance management for the prison health system to provide the same quality of health service as received by the general public
How were resource needs met?	From April 2003, the Department of Health is responsible for funding prison healthcare. It has been made clear in the action plan the resource implications of every health issue improvement. The key issue was to ensure that the existing resources were used efficiently and effectively
Step 4: Action planning	
Summary of the action planning process	The action plan and health improvement and modernisation programme for prisoners was signed by Durham and Chester le Street PCT chief executive and the prison governors. Key tasks were to: improve workforce development, staff training and continuing professional development; improving services such as primary care management, clinical governance, mental health, suicide and self-harm management; substance misuse; reception screening; health promotion; dental services; pharmacy services; infectious diseases; health information system; and improving facilities and services specific to women prisoners. All proposals for action were identified and designated to lead key individuals. The date for completion of tasks and performance measures was identified for every action plan

Case study 2: Health needs assessment within Durham cluster of prisons	
Step 5: Moving on/review	
How well was the action plan implemented?	The priorities mentioned were identified for implementation by a newly appointed prison health development manager
What was achieved by the project?	Priorities were identified and some changes to improve and redesign services implemented to set the example that services could improve within a custodial environment and make resources more cost effective
How did it contribute to reducing inequalities?	A high proportion of prisoners come from socially excluded sections of the community
What was learned through the project's successes and challenges?	Involving stakeholders and key professionals in assessing prisoners' unmet needs and providing effective healthcare to them while in custody, even for a short period, can make a significant contribution to the health of individuals
What needs to happen next?	Very important to keep prison steering group meetings going to involve key stakeholders and professionals in improving prison healthcare services
What main message from the last HNA will you take forward to the next?	HNA within prison could be extensively improved, but the main message was the importance of close cooperation between prison healthcare and NHS (PCT) staff

Source: Cavanagh and Chadwick (2005)

Discussion Task

Suppose you have been asked to do a HNA amongst prisoners, what might be the main health and well-being issues of interest? Where would you get this information (sources)?

Comments: (a) Marginalised community—deprived, financial, educational, housing, etc. (b) Health-lifestyle issues (drinking, smoking exercise, obesity), mental health (depression, anxiety, schizophrenia, psychosis), drug and alcohol issues. (c) Information sources—national literature (other prison HNA findings), prison sources (disease registers, case note reviews, healthcare service activity data), corporate (questionnaires, interviews, don't forget the prison healthcare team).

Challenges in Conducting Health Needs Assessments

Although HNAs have a structured approach, conducting them in practice is not as straightforward. Part of the problem is definitional. Need, as has been pointed out, is a complex concept and understood differently by different people. The HNA team will be tasked to develop a shared language between stakeholders. Another difficulty lies in the type of need that is measured. Most needs assessments use proxies (e.g. service usage statistics) for need and this may not be an accurate estimation of real need.

Not all populations are easily reached (e.g. homeless people, vulnerable migrants, gypsies and travellers, and sex workers injecting drug users, socially excluded groups, undocumented immigrants) and sometimes, access may require careful negotiation and innovative approaches. Especially where a corporate approach is taken to the HNA, there may be difficulties in engaging different groups within the community and ensuring an appropriate balance of 'voices' across the spectrum of stakeholders.

Many HNAs rely on existing data as collecting primary data can be costly and time consuming. Accessing robust data may be problematic, particularly where the population is too small to allow statistically valid estimates to be generated. Expertise may also be lacking in the range of data collection methods that are needed to collect and analyse the data.

Services have different priorities and it can be challenging securing a consensus on what the most important priorities emerging from the HNA are. What constitutes a priority may also be perceived differently by the lay public and professionals.

Working across organisational and professional boundaries can represent a big shift for the staff involved in the HNA. Senior level commitment to the process and particularly to implementing the necessary changes is vital. If the HNA takes a long time to complete, it is common for team impetus and commitment to be strong at the start but wane over time.

Finally, it is essential that the findings of the needs assessment are translated into effective, sustainable action and that the resulting changes are evaluated. However many HNAs that have been undertaken fall short of the full cycle (i.e. steps 1–5). One reason for this is that the assembled team may have good population profiling and data analysis skills but is lacking in the area of action planning, making change and evaluation. Other factors may be a lack of resources to deliver the full HNA or inability to sustain the commitment of senior people over the entire process.

Joint Strategic Needs Assessment

A fairly recent addition to the armoury of needs assessment is the joint strategic needs assessment (JSNA). As a requirement of the Local Government and Public Involvement in Health Act 2007, Primary Care Trusts (now replaced by Clinical Commissioning Groups) and local authorities were mandated to develop JSNAs of the health and well-being of their local communities. The JSNA describes a process that identifies current and future health and well-being needs in light of existing services, and informs future service planning taking into account evidence of effectiveness (Department of Health 2007, p. 7). It sets out an over-arching assessment of community needs and establishes a shared, evidence-based consensus on key local priorities which informs the strategic direction of service delivery to tackle those priorities, improve outcomes and reduce health inequalities. It is therefore an important tool in service planning and commissioning. The elements of JSNA are illustrated in Fig. 5.

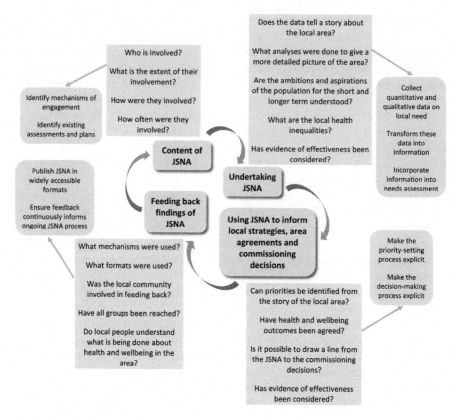

Fig. 5 The Joint Strategic Needs Assessment (JSNA) process (*Source*: Department of Health 2007)

A simplistic view of JSNA is that it represents a scaling up or escalation of HNA in order to see the big picture. Indeed, JSNA is similar to HNA in terms of (a) assessing health need, (b) maintaining the focus on health inequalities and (c) being underpinned by partnership working, community engagement and evidence of effectiveness. However, there are some key differences.

JSNA is a *strategic* process: it scans the whole population not just a subgroup, and assesses not only current, but future need. With JSNA, need is assessed over a period of 3–5 years, but it can include a longer term assessment (5–10 years) to take account of changes in structural factors such as demography. JSNA is also a *continuous* and *iterative* process of collating and sharing data, refining the analyses at each cycle and enhancing understanding of the new data. JSNA is unique to each local area and provides a broader context and evidence base for all other needs assessments.

Another significant characteristic of JSNA is that it is *joined-up*, enabling assessment to be conducted across organisational and sector boundaries in a unified way. The underpinning logic is that population needs span health and social care spheres and tackling those needs requires multisectoral action, for example, the coordinated provision of services for long term conditions, and joined up approaches to obesity, nutrition and physical activity. If these different sectors can jointly shape their planning and delivery, then they will be better able to secure integrated and more effective provision across a range of services.

In order to deliver this challenging objective, it is essential to have an understanding of the needs of the population and the wider determinants of health from several different but joined up perspectives. The introduction of JSNA thus marked a major change in the way in which the Department of Health required the NHS, local authorities and other strategic partners to consider the needs of their local populations and in how they respond with effective commissioning of services to address those needs.

The three core functions of the JSNA can be summarised as follows:

• Provide data analysis profiling the health and well-being status of local communities.
• Identify where inequalities exist.
• Use local community views and evidence of effectiveness of interventions to shape the future investment and disinvestments of services.

Currently, the JSNA is co-produced by the Directors of Public Health, Adult Social Services and Children's Services in a local area. Ultimately, it is not about the production of a document but about local authorities, the NHS and other key partners working together to establish an over-arching, evidence-based consensus on local health and well-being priorities.

Conclusion

HNA, or more appropriately health and well-being needs assessment (HWBNA), is one of a range of approaches available to practitioners and commissioners across all sectors to inform decision-making processes. An understanding of HNA requires a clear definition of need, which from a public health perspective implies the capacity to benefit from an intervention. The starting point for conducting a HNA is the population of interest. The five principal steps in the process are: (a) agree aims, objectives and project framework; (b) identify and assess population health priorities; (c) assess a priority for action; (d) action planning for change and (e) review/ evaluation. The process involves engagement with the target population, and a multi-agency approach to assessment, planning and implementation of programmes to ensure that appropriate cross-sectoral actions are taken on the findings. Outputs from HNA can be used to inform other forms of assessment (HEA, HIA and IIA), as well as regional and local policy documents.

References

Bradshaw, J. R. (1972). The taxonomy of social need. In G. McLachlan (Ed.), *Problems and progress in medical care*. Oxford: Oxford University Press.

Bradshaw, J. (1994). The conceptualisation and measurement of need: A social policy perspective. In J. Popay & G. Williams (Eds.), *Researching the people's health* (pp. 45–57). London: Routledge.

Cavanagh, S., & Chadwick, K. (2005). *Health needs assessment: A practical guide*. London: National Institute for Health and Clinical Excellence.

Dahlgren, G., & Whitehead, M. (1991). *Policies and strategies to promote social equity in health*. Stockholm: Institute for Future Studies.

Department of Health. (2007). *Guidance on joint strategic needs assessment*. London: DoH.

Elkheir, R. (2007). *Health needs assessment: A practical approach*. Retrieved September 29, 2015, from http://www.sjph.net.sd/files/vol2i2p81-88.pdf.

Hooper, J., & Longworth, P. (2002). *Health needs assessment workbook*. London: Health Development Agency.

Powell, J. (2006). *Health needs assessment: A systematic approach*. London: National Library for Health.

Quigley, R., Cavanagh, S., Harrison, D., Taylor, L., & Pottle, M. (2005). *Clarifying approaches to assessment: Health needs assessment, health impact assessment, integrated impact assessment, health equity audit, and race equality impact assessment*. London: Health Development Agency.

Rogers, C., & Fox, R. (2005). *Health needs assessment*. Wales: National Public Health Service for Wales.

Stevens, A., & Gillam, S. (1998). Needs assessment: From theory to practice. *British Medical Journal, 316*, 1448–1452.

Stevens, A., & Rafferty, J. (1994, 1997). *Health care needs assessment: The epidemiologically based needs assessment reviews*. Vol. 1 and 2. Oxford: Radcliffe Medical Press.

Stevens, A. J., & Rafferty, J. (1997). *Health care needs assessment*. Oxford: Radcliffe.

Stevens, A., Raftery, J., Mant, J., & Simpson, S. (2004). *Health care needs assessment: The epidemiologically based needs assessment reviews* (Vol. 1 and 2). Oxford: Radcliffe Medical Press.

Williams, R., & Wright, J. (1998). Epidemiological issues in health needs assessment. *British Medical Journal, 316*, 1379–1382.

Wright, J. (2001). Assessing health needs. In D. Pencheon (Ed.), *Oxford handbook of public health practice*. Oxford: Oxford University Press.

Recommended Reading

Cavanagh, S., & Chadwick, K. (2005). *Health needs assessment: A practical guide*. London: National Institute for Health and Clinical Excellence.

Hooper, J., & Longworth, P. (2002). *Health needs assessment workbook*. London: Health Development Agency.

Department of Health. (2007). *Guidance on joint strategic needs assessment*. London: DoH.

Quigley, R., Cavanagh, S., Harrison, D., Taylor, L., & Pottle, M. (2005). *Clarifying approaches to assessment: Health needs assessment, health impact assessment, integrated impact assessment, health equity audit, and race equality impact assessment*. London: Health Development Agency.

Demography in Public Health Intelligence

Ivan Gee and Krishna Regmi

Abstract Demography is the scientific study of human population. For the last few decades, demographic models and methods have been frequently used to analyse or measure the births, deaths and migration within human populations. Public health practitioners and public health analysts regularly require information about health demography, which deals with the contents and methods of demography within the context of health and healthcare. In other words, health demography deals with the demographic attributes that may influence or concern health status and health behaviour, as well as the health-related phenomena which influence the demographic attributes of the population (Pol and Thomas 2013). Following an overview of health demography, this chapter will discuss the nature and extent of public health problems within the context of present and future patterns of demographic change. This chapter will also highlight some applications, concepts and methods related to health.

After reading this chapter you should be able to:

- Define the concept and meaning of populations
- Discuss the nature and extent of public health problems within the context of present and future patterns of demographic change
- Examine sources of population data and their strengths and weaknesses.

I. Gee (✉)
Center for Public Health, Liverpool John Moores University,
Henry Cotton Building, 15-21 Webster St, Liverpool L3 2ET, UK
e-mail: i.l.gee@ljmu.ac.uk

K. Regmi
Faculty of Health and Social Sciences, University of Bedfordshire,
Putteridge Bury Campus, IHR-32, Luton LU2 8LE, UK
e-mail: Krishna.regmi@beds.ac.uk

© Springer International Publishing Switzerland 2016
K. Regmi, I. Gee (eds.), *Public Health Intelligence*,
DOI 10.1007/978-3-319-28326-5_10

187

Introduction

While accessing and analysing any public health problems, we often look at the population who are mostly at risk of exposure to potential risk factors. In gathering evidence we might examine how large the population is, what are the magnitude of health problems, stratifying by age, sex and location and we might need to know the dynamics of the population.

Demography is the science of population or the scientific study of human population, and it is concerned with the analysis of population size and structure with reference to its three determinants: fertility, mortality and migration. As the London School of Economics argues (LSE 2014), demography relates to social and policy issues, as well as population growth globally and the challenges faced due to ageing populations, as well as the potential implications of migration (in and out) among populations which are closely interlinked; for example, fewer children will bring some pressures on care and cost implications for pensioners and older populations.

Pol and Thomas (2013) note that health demography as a discipline 'involves the application of the content and methods of demography to the study of health and healthcare' (p. 1). They suggest that 'health demography concerns itself with the manner in which demographic attributes influence both the health status and health behaviour of populations, and how, in turn, health-related phenomenon affect demographic attributes' (p. 1). From that point of view, we can say that health demography reflects some characteristics of biostatistics and epidemiology considers the health aspects at both levels of health—individual-level (clinical medicine) and population-level (social epidemiology).

Generally, as Pol and Thomas (2013, pp. 1–4) suggest, we can view demography from the different broader perspectives—epidemiology, sociology, anthropology, geography and economics, and each discipline has some link to the study of health and healthcare. Assessing health and disease through measuring mortality and morbidity is a core aspect of demographical disciplines. Population size, composition and distribution are major attributes which help to understand the level of health service access and utilisation, as well as demand.

Epidemiology: particularly social epidemiology, deals with the distribution of illness within the population and recognises that disease or illness is caused by different social behaviours or dynamics of different social groups.

Sociology: deals with the study of society or organisation; in this case focussing on the organisation of healthcare. Similarly, cultural similarities and differences have roles in healthcare organisations.

Medical geography: considers the spatial distribution of various health-related phenomena that involve disease, health conditions, health professionals and healthcare organisations.

Economics in health: (or health economics) is a well-established field which measures the level of healthcare in terms of costs at the system, practitioner and consumer levels.

It can therefore be argued that demography is a large discipline which has good links in terms of assessing, analysing and developing appropriate actions within health or public health.

Discussion Task
What are the uses of demography in public health?

Comments: Decision-makers and policy-planners will use demographic profiles to identify and characterise health problems in the community. They will be able to assess the healthcare needs of the population that might help in planning, prioritising and implementation using appropriate and available resources, which ultimately address the aim of public health—to control and prevent health problems. At the same time it is important to note that studying different socio-economic and political determinants will help to identify the underpinning factors responsible for the occurrence of disease or illness (Mendoza et al. 1999, p. 68).

Grundy and Murphy (2015, p. 735) pointed out that 'health and healthcare needs of a population cannot be measured or met without knowledge of its size and characteristics'. Public health is concerned with health of the general public, which depends upon the dynamic relationship between the numbers of people, the space which they occupy and the skill that they have acquired in providing for their needs. Several demographic factors, or foci, are then important in supporting our understanding of public health:

- Population size and its change over time (growth or decline)
- The composition of the population (or its structure: age, ethnicity, etc.)
- Distribution of population in space
  (from Park 2011)

Discussion Task
How do these three foci then relate to assessing the health problems of the population?

Comment: There are three important foci of the demography—population size, population composition or structure, and distribution of population. In relation to public health, you might have explored how these would affect potential diseases or associated risks looking at 'person', 'place' and 'time' attributes: How many and what sorts of people are affected (person), where do problems arise (place) and when do they arise (time).

It is important that understanding of population dynamics always appears as a core element for estimating future population size and structure that should provide a guide for healthcare planning and management (Grundy and Murphy 2015). Therefore demography supports in our seeking responses to the problems or questions about how and why the health of populations change, what possible consequences may result, and how these could be measured. In addition, this will help in understanding the causes and consequences of disease, levels of health status, attributes and beliefs towards access to and utilisation of health services, health professionals' behaviours and health outcomes (Pol and Thomas 2013, p. 1).

Discussion Task
Consider what demographic or health data has been collected about you/your family and your community in the last few years? And why are you interested?

Comment: You might have considered data related to births, death, morbidity, childhood, environment and lifestyle, healthcare, economy, etc. Information on how large the population is and what it is comprised of (children/adult/elderly or male/female) and where they are found (urban/rural).

Global Population Trends: Issues and Challenges

In the 1970s when the authors of this chapter were children there were less than 4 billion people in the world. By the time we finished university in the 1990s there were over 5 billion and by 2010 there were nearly 7 billion. Projections suggest the global population will reach at least 9 billion by 2050 (US Census Bureau 2010). The global population has steadily increased since 1960 and will have more than doubled in less than 50 years. Figure 1 shows the rate of global population change since 1970.

Clearly any increase in the total global population places strain on the world's ability to support that number of people. As the number of people increases we need to provide more food, more housing, more schools, more healthcare, etc. Many commentators have speculated that there will be a finite limit to the capacity of the globe to support the population. Perhaps the earliest of these was Thomas Malthus (1766–1834) who suggested that while unchecked population growth is exponential while the growth of the food supply was expected to be arithmetical (i.e. linear).

Malthus then predicted that sooner or later a famine and disease would curb the population—a Malthusian catastrophe. Malthus and later Malthusian thinkers believed that cycles of exponential population growth would be curbed by Malthusian catastrophes, unless society controlled populations. Malthus believed in self-control as a means to control procreation, later neo-Malthusians have advocated extensive birth control and modern China can be viewed as an example of these Malthusian approaches in practice (see 'Case Study: China's One-Child Policy').

Fig. 1 Global population
change (*Source*: US
Census Bureau 2011)

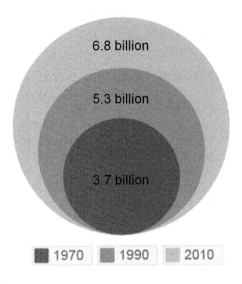

Case Study: China's One-Child Policy

Since 1980 China has enforced a policy that limits couples (with some exceptions and exemptions for ethnic minorities) to a single child. Prior to this previous Chinese administrations had encouraged couples to have children to increase the workforce. But by the 1970s it was clear that the rates of population growth were not sustainable. The policy operates by providing incentives for those who adhere to the policy, such as increased access to education, childcare and healthcare, and penalties for those who did not comply, e.g. removal of benefits, fines and sterilisations. The policy has been enforced strictly in urban areas but has been harder to control in rural populations. The birth rate in China has reduced considerably over the period of the policy which was slightly relaxed in 2013. China now has an ageing population and there are some concerns that the working population will not be large enough to support the gradually ageing population.

More recent commentators have highlighted the ability of the world to accommodate increased numbers without Malthusian collapses. We have developed more intensive agriculture, better crop strains, new techniques, etc. that have allowed us to support substantial population growth, but increasingly the consensus is that there will be a finite capacity for human populations that will be limited by environmental factors other than just food production. Population growth is now slowing in the vast majority of countries outside Sub-Saharan Africa and projections suggest that it is likely that the global population will hit peak at 8–10.5 billion in the period 2050–2070. By 2100 there is an 80 % chance that the population will be between 6.2 and 11.1 billion (EEA 2012).

Discussion Task
Do you have any idea how many people live in a given place at a given time?

Comment: Though this question seems very simple, the process of getting an accurate answer involves careful definitions of time, place and person (TPP), and the use of carefully worked-out methods for securing the most accurate information. Getting accurate information on numbers requires suitable counts, but all counts are likely to miss certain types of people in the population, who are not present on official registers such as the electoral role or GP lists (e.g. homeless, illegal immigrants). As a public health student/practitioner, we need to know whether the present number is smaller or larger than it was in the past, and what this number would likely be at some time in the future (i.e. in terms of rates and trends).

Types of Demography

The study of population may vary, but the important types are briefly discussed here:

1. **Formal demography**: is considered as a mathematical measure which deals with the demographic processes which can be summarized as:

   - Fertility (crude birth rate, general fertility rate, age-specific birth rate)
   - Mortality (crude death rate, infant/neonatal mortality rate, age/cause-specific mortality)
   - Migration (in-out migration, age/race-specific migration)
     (Farmer et al. n.d.)

2. **Social demography**: deals with the 'determinants and consequences of population size, distribution and composition and of the demographic processes of fertility, mortality and migration that determine them' (Murdock and Ellis 1991, p. 4).

3. **Applied demography**: refers to the 'production, dissemination and analysis of demographic information' and that helps in 'planning and reporting the study of population size, spatial distribution and composition' (Rives and Serow 1984, p. 9).

These different approaches all require information about populations and how they are changing. This information is delivered through use of the tools discussed in the next section.

Tools of Demography

Mendoza et al. (1999) note that while studying the foci of the demography (population size, composition and distribution), we need to deal with the numbers, and these would be in the form of counts, rates and ratios/proportions.

Counts, Rates and Ratios

Counts: simply measure the absolute number of any demographic events (births, deaths disease, etc.) occurring in a defined population in a specific time-frame. This provides us with the raw numbers, e.g. how many births there are at any one time/place. This is useful but cannot tell us much about how these events might vary between different places and areas, as the different areas will all have different population sizes.

Rate: is the frequency of occurrence of events over a given time period/interval for a particular population size. It 'measures the amount of change' for a specified population size (Mendoza et al. 1999, p. 72). Rates are useful while measuring the events, for example, new cases of disease—incidence rate (number of events occurring within a given time interval divided by the number of population members who are exposed to risk or illness during the same time interval (see chapter 'Types of Data and Measures of Disease', section 'Part I: Understanding data sources'). Because the size of the populations in different areas are is accounted for rates allow crude comparisons between areas. These are called crude rates as although they account for differences in population size, they don't account for other differences such as the relative ages of the populations.

Ratio: is considered as a single number that refers to the relative size of two attributes; for example, if you divide 'C' by 'D' times K $(=C/D \times K)$ (where K is a population size factor which may be the value of 100 or 1000 or 10,000 or 100,000. It tells us what the ratio is per 1000 or 10,000 population, etc.). In this example, the value of 'C' and 'D' will define the numerator and denominator, respectively, for a specific geographic area and period of time.

Generally, in a ratio the value of C (numerator) may or may not be a part of the D (denominator); for example, a sex ratio, i.e. number of males/number of females times 100.

Proportion is a type of ratio often used in public health measures. While measuring proportion, the numerator is part of the denominator. In the given example, if we are to compute proportion then we simply divide C by $C + D$ times K. When K is equal to 100, the value of the proportion will be expressed as a percentage.

Discussion Task
What sort of things do we want to know about a population when considering factors that might influence health?

Comments: Factors you considered might include

- Size
- Age structure
- Fertility
- Ethnic mix
- Education
- Socio-economic distribution
- Projected changes—fertility, mortality, mobility, marriage
- Population pyramids

We hope you have already understood the value of counts, rates, ratios and proportions. In health demography, an effective means of describing the age and sex composition of the population in a graphical representation is the population pyramid (sometimes known as a 'demographic tree'). Population pyramids are a simple way of displaying the structure of a population. In these particular examples, the bars are numbers to show the difference in the **absolute size** of populations (but proportions can also be used).

To develop the pyramid, first you need to compute either the absolute number or percentage of the population for each age-sex group. Each age-group (usually 5 year age bands) is represented by a horizontal bar (generally the youngest population will be at the base of the pyramid), males are traditionally represented on the left side of the central vertical axis with females to the right, and the length of each bar refers to the size (absolute number or percentage %) of the population (Mendoza et al. 1999, p. 77). It therefore demonstrates the relative sizes of specific age and sex groups—see the examples of the population pyramids for four different countries below.

Discussion Task

1. What can you tell about pyramid Fig. 2 (size, age structure, fertility, mortality).
2. What could you guess from this about the health needs of these populations?

Comments: This country has a high fertility rate (lots of births), the largest numbers are in the 0–4 age band, and not many are living through to maturity; life expectancy is poor, as emphasised by the concave shape of the pyramid. This suggests a less economically developed country, e.g. Sub-Saharan Africa.

Health needs will be considerable, maternal and infant care needs improving, vaccination rates are likely to be low, healthcare is likely to be limited in general. However due to the early mortality facilities for the elderly, e.g. to tackle diseases such as stroke and dementia are not likely to be extensively needed.

Discussion Task

What can you tell about pyramid Fig. 3 (size, age structure, fertility, mortality)?

Comments: This is a much larger population; the birth rate is still high but is decreasing and mortality is also high but is delayed compared to Fig. 1, numbers do not start decreasing till age 15–19 suggesting that birth infant mortality is lower, e.g. India.

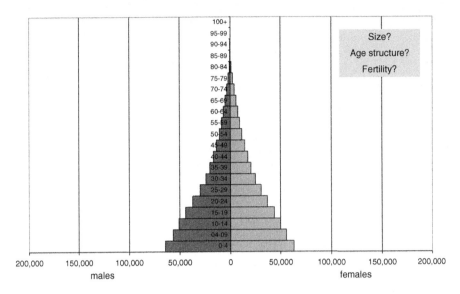

Fig. 2 Population pyramid a)

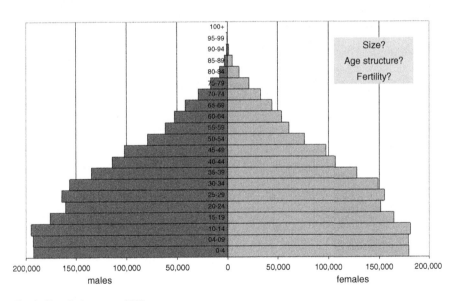

Fig. 3 Population pyramid b)

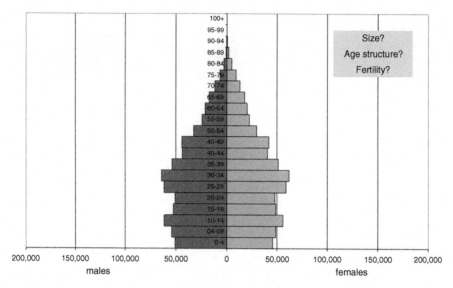

Fig. 4 Population pyramid c)

Discussion Task

What can you tell about pyramid Fig. 4 (size, age structure and fertility)?

Comments: This shows a clear reduction in the birth rate (there are fewer 0–4 s than there are 30–34 year olds for example). This might be the effect of a country like China's one-child policy. There is little variation in the size of the population in each age-group, and life expectancy is good compared to Sub-Saharan Africa. However, relatively small numbers have lived into their 50s which suggests that conditions were not so good in this country in the last 50 years, so it's not a country which has been developed for a long period.

Discussion Task

What can you tell about pyramid Fig. 5 (size, age structure and fertility)? Can you discuss some key significance from a public health point of view?

Comments: This is a typical classical shape of a mature or more economically developed society, where the practice of having no children or smaller families, i.e. low fertility rates, has been the norm for several generations. Life expectancy is very good with a large proportion of the population living to later in life (e.g. Europe).

In public health practice—particularly in public health planning and decision-making, we need to identify and characterise health problems of the community in terms of how large the problem is and who are the most affected population in order to plan, prioritise and implement the public health interventions appropriately. As you will be aware, the ultimate aim of the public health work is to be able to control, manage and prevent health problems.

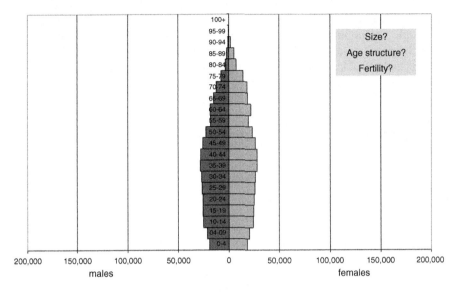

Fig. 5 Population pyramid d)

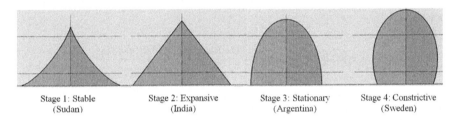

Fig. 6 Population pyramid shapes across the demographic transition

The pyramids in Figs. 2–5 demonstrate the range of population distributions that we can see around the world today and back into the past. They form a progression from high birth rate and early mortality through to very low birth rates and later mortality. These can be classified into 4 stages as summarised in Fig. 6, and form the basis of the so-called **demographic transition** model. This model suggests that as countries become more developed and move from poorer rural economies to wealthier industrialised economies then the population distribution changes as birth rates reduce and average mortality recedes to later in life.

Stage 1. Stable: very high birth rates are offset by high death rates relatively early in life, including high infant and childhood mortality, resulting in a relatively stable or slowly growing population, e.g. Sudan.

Stage 2. Expansive: birth rates are still high but improved circumstances such as childhood vaccinations, improved sanitation and primary healthcare are reducing death rates, particularly early in life. This results in a rapidly growing population, e.g. India.

Stage 3. Stationary: birth rates are reducing and deaths tend to come later in life. People are confident that their children are likely to survive, so they don't need such large families. Good healthcare and environmental improvements are delaying deaths to older ages. The population continues to grow but the growth rate is slowing, e.g. Argentina.

Stage 4. Constrictive: birth rates are very low, frequently much less than two births per woman and deaths are on average delayed to older ages. The population is shrinking due to the low birth rate and will on average be ageing, e.g. Sweden.

Dependency Ratios

The consequence of having high birth rates (Stage 1. High fertility countries) or low death rates (Stage 4 countries) is that the number of very young or elderly people in the population will be high. This places considerable strain on a country's resources as these groups are not working, so not contributing to the economy and they have high demands on society, e.g. for schooling or healthcare. The balance between these dependents (children under 15 and adults over 65) and the working population (people between 15 and 65) is the dependency ratio, and is generally presented as a percentage.

$$\text{Dependency ratio}\,(\%) = \frac{\text{Dependent population} \times 100}{\text{Working population}}$$

Discussion Task

Why would governments need to know about dependency ratios? What does a rising dependency ratio mean for a government?

Comments: Governments need to monitor dependency ratios as changes in this will have implications for things like the productivity of the economy and the services required to support the dependents. This will be different for populations with high dependency due to high birth rates compared to countries like the UK with increasing dependency due to an ageing population.

An increasing dependency ratio would mean a greater responsibility was placed upon governments to ensure that the basic needs of all its citizens are met and it would require governments to invest more heavily in social infrastructure. Many European countries including the UK have ageing populations that are requiring greater investment in health and social care facilities. Much of the current concern for the NHS is based on the strains being placed on services due to a population that is living for longer. In rapidly developing countries such as India, while there has been a marked reduction in birth rates there remains a legacy of previously high birth rates and the successes of improved child and maternal health care (such as vaccination programmes). This has resulted in a relatively young population placing pressures on areas such as schools, housing, employment and infrastructure. Young populations are also associated with risk of social unrest, particularly where unemployment is high and people don't feel they can move on in society. This has been termed the **youth bulge** and is associated with the unrest that has been seen in North African states and the uprisings of the Arab Spring during 2010–2011.

Sources of Population Data

The most common sources of demographic data are census, sample surveys and registration systems (Mendoza et al. 1999). In the UK, three potential sources are:

1. **Office for National Statistics (ONS)**

   - 2011 census
   - Mid-year estimates
   - Sub-national population projections

2. **General practice**

   - Registered population
   - Exeter registered resident
   - Strategic tracing service

3. **Local authorities**

   - Electoral roll
   - School rolls
   - Local planning data

Discussion Task
Consider local authority data sources, and review how this source would be useful to public health bodies when considering new development (e.g. a new hospital)

Comments: The sources available at a local authority level (district/provincial estimates and projections), which are able to help local public health or environmental health planners, are able to provide detail on proposed developments. The electoral roll can be useful for picking up possible population growth not identified by other sources, and generally they are considered more accurate than the figures from the Office for National Statistics (ONS) for planning purposes. However, it is difficult to gather truly representative information from these populations; for example, homeless people, travellers, illegal immigrants, unregistered migrant workers and 'special populations' — armed forces and dependants, or prisoners, tend not to be included on formal registers such as the electoral roll or on GP lists. ONS estimates try to account for these missing populations and are regularly updated to account for in and out migration, but these remain estimates.

Conclusion

Public health is concerned with populations because health in the group depends upon the dynamics and relationships between the number of people, the space which they occupy, and the skills they have acquired in providing for their healthcare needs. The importance of this knowledge for more rational health programme planning, management and evaluation cannot be overemphasised. This chapter explored the main types of demography and how global populations have changed over the last 50 years. It highlights how demographic information can be presented using population pyramids and what these can tell us about the nature of populations and how they change. We have also identified that the most important sources of demographic information are censuses, surveys and registration systems. The less popular sources include voters, school rosters and others.

References

European Environment Agency. (2012). *World population projections—IIASA probabilistic projections compared to UN projections*. Retrieved September 18, 2015, from http://www.eea. europa.eu/data-and-maps/figures/world-population-projections-iiasa-probabilistic.

Farmer, F., Moon, Z., & Miller, W. (n.d.). *Understanding community demographics*. Retrieved June 6, 2015, from http://ruralsoc.uark.edu/pubs/Understanding%20Community%20 DemographicsPDF.pdf.

Gray, A. (2001). *World health and disease*. Buckingham, England: Open University Press.

Grundy, E., & Murphy, M. (2015). Demography and public health. In R. Detels, M. Gulliford, Q. Abdool Karim, & T. C. Chuan (Eds.), *Oxford textbook of global public health* (6th ed.). Oxford: Oxford University Press.

Lee, K., Buse, K., & Fustukian, S. (2002). *Health policy in a globalising world*. Cambridge, England: Cambridge University Press.

London School of Economics. (2014). Demography and health. Retrieved September 18, 2015, from http://www.lse.ac.uk/LSEHealthAndSocialCare/research/LSEHealth/DemographyandHealth. aspx.

Mendoza, O. M., Borja, M. P., Sevilla, T. L., Ancheta, C. A., Saniel, O. P., et al. (1999). *Foundations of statistical analysis for the health sciences*. Paranaque, Philippines: Camins Printing Press.

Murdock, S., & Ellis, D. (1991). *Applied demography*. Boulder, CO: Westview Press.

Park, K. (2011). *Park's textbook of preventative and social medicine*. Jabalpur, India: MS Banarsidas Bhanot.

Pol, L. G., & Thomas, R. K. (2013). *The demography of health and healthcare*. New York: Springer.

Rives, N., & Serow, W. (1984). *Introduction to applied demography: data sources and estimation techniques*. Beverly Hills, LA: Sage.

United Nations. (2012). *The millennium development goals report 2012*. New York: UN. Retrieved September 18, 2015, from http://www.un.org/millenniumgoals/pdf/MDG%20Report%20 2012.pdf.

Bureau, U. S. C. (2010). *Global population projections*. Retrieved September 18, 2015, from https://www.census.gov/population/international/data/idb/worldpopgraph.php.

Recommended Reading

Davis, S. (2012). *Chapter 1: Demography*. In: Chief Medical Officers Report 2011. London: Department of Health.

Hoque, N., McGehee, M. A., & Bradshaw, B. S. (2013). *Applied demography and public health*. New York: Springer.

Leone, T. (2010). How can demography inform health policy? *Health Economics, Policy and Law, 5*, 1–11.

Data Presentation

Julian Flowers and Katie Johnson

Abstract This chapter will address key issues in the presentation of data in public health intelligence. Data needs to be communicated to create insight, or influence change and the visualisation and presentation of data in public health practice is a core skill and growing in importance. It will show how to select and create appropriate charts, discuss some of the new and developing tools available, and give some examples of how data can influence policy and practice and visualisation can bring insight and clarity.

After reading this chapter you will be able to:

- Describe the importance of effective data presentation and the key considerations when choosing how to present the data.
- Understand the different types of data presentation, their strengths and limitations, and when they are best used.
- Know the key principles and common pitfalls of data presentation.
- Understand the benefits of interactive data visualisation and how different techniques can be used to enhance data presentation.
- Know where to go to find further reading and tools that may help you present your data.

The Importance of Effective Data Presentation

Getting Your Message Across

Data is the lifeblood of public health practice. It underpins policy and practice and effective data presentation is a core skill. This is more than drawing graphs—it is communicating what data says, why it says what it says and what to do about it.

J. Flowers (✉)
Knowledge and Intelligence Service, Public Health England,
West Wing, Victoria House, Capital Park, Cambridge CB21 5XB, UK
e-mail: Julian.flowers@phe.gov.uk

K. Johnson
Norfolk and Norwich University Hospitals NHS Foundation Trust (on behalf of Health Education East of England), Colney Lane, Norwich NR4 7UY, UK
e-mail: katie.johnson3@nhs.net

© Springer International Publishing Switzerland 2016
K. Regmi, I. Gee (eds.), *Public Health Intelligence*,
DOI 10.1007/978-3-319-28326-5_11

This is not to say that drawing charts is not important—we need to select the right charts for the job and present them in the right way (generally less is more). There is an increasing evidence base on how to present data and an emergent discipline of data visualisation (vizzing) and creating infographics.

Visualising quantitative data can enable understanding of far more complex information than other means of communication.

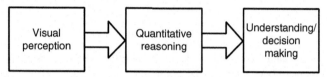

There are well known examples of how data has been used to influence policy or public health. For example, John Snow's classic maps of the distribution of cholera in 1850s Soho helped identify the source of the outbreak and the public health intervention which hastened its end (removal of the Broad Street pump handle).

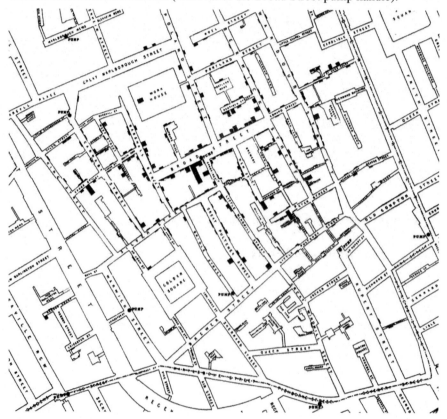

Source: https://upload.wikimedia.org/wikipedia/commons/thumb/2/27/Snow-cholera-map-1.jpg/600px-Snow-cholera-map-1.jpg

Florence Nightingale created a new chart type—coxcomb diagrams, sometimes known as Nightingale's Rose, to highlight that the plight of soldiers in the Crimean war was largely due to conditions in the military hospitals not the battlefield.

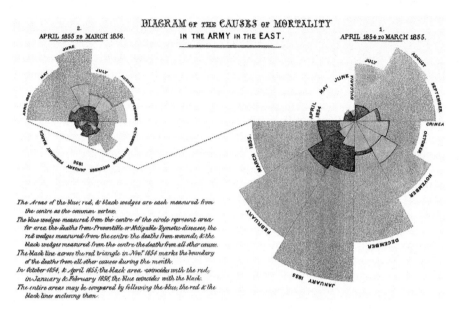

Source:https://upload.wikimedia.org/wikipedia/commons/thumb/1/17/Nightingale-mortality.jpg/440px-Nightingale-mortality.jpg

To illustrate some of the points in this chapter we'll use some data published in the Guardian newspaper about death rates following elective surgery for aortic aneurysms.

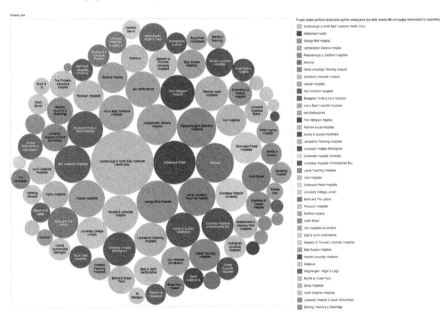

Source: created by the author from http://www.theguardian.com/news/datablog/2010/jun/13/abdominal-aorticaneurysm-surgery-statistics

This chart was published as part of the Guardian data blog (http://www.theguardian.com/news/datablog/2010/jun/13/abdominal-aortic-aneurysm-surgery-statistics).

It is known a bubble plot and it aims to show the elective mortality rate for surgical repair of aortic aneurysms in NHS Trusts in England.

What messages is the chart trying to get across: what does it actually show? how could it be improved?

Transparency and Open Data

Increasingly governments are putting more data into the public domain and encouraging the public sector to do the same. The belief is that opening up data will improve public accountability, inform choice and improve quality. The latest initiative in the health sector in England is MyNHS, which brings together public health data alongside performance data for providers and commissioners. This can be accessed at http://www.nhs.uk/Service-Search/performance/search and a screen shot of the home page is shown below. You can search the site for data about services or health in your area (within England).

My NHS *BETA* | Data for better services   NHS Choices >

Performance information to support transparency and drive quality

Making our data transparent will help to drive up quality and create even better services.

Here you can see key data used by the NHS and local councils to monitor performance and shape the services you use. We'll continually add to the information, listen to what you want, and work to make it as clear as possible.

We want your feedback on the contents and presentation of this site, whether you are a care professional, clinician, manager, carer or a member of the public.

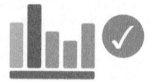

Explore the data

 Hospitals
View quality indicator information on NHS hospitals (private-sector providers not included)

 Social care
See how local authorities perform on provision of adult social services

 Public health services
Get data on how public health services delivered by hospitals and general practices perform within local authority areas

 Public health outcomes
The NHS works with local authorities to protect and improve public health. See key public health outcomes in each local authority area

 Mental health hospitals
View quality indicator information for mental health hospitals provided by NHS Trusts

 General practice
See a range of quality indicator information for general practice

 Consultants
See consultant outcome data for a range of specialties

Also available on NHS Choices

 Care providers
Search for information about care homes and care at home services

How is data presented within this tool? how easy is it to get information about your local hospital or general practice?

> **Discussion Task**
> Discuss in a group the potential benefits and issues with making health and public health information accessible to the public.

Choosing the Type of Presentation

When choosing how to present your data, the first step is to consider what you are trying to say. Think about the story you want to tell with the information and the key messages you want your audience to understand. This will help you to choose which data to present and how best to present it. You may find it useful to write a research question for each figure or table. For example, "How have premature cardiovascular mortality rates in London changed over the past 10 years?" Or "In Lancashire, is there a relationship between general practice performance of blood pressure control and deprivation?" By stating your key question, it focuses exactly which data you need to present and the key messages your visualisation must portray.

The next step is to define and understand your audience. Who is the target audience and who else may use your data presentation? Think about what they already know about the topic, what they may be interested in and what data interpretation skills they may have. A data presentation won't be used if it's not of interest to the audience and it must be easily understandable.

Once you have defined your key messages, considered your audience and therefore chosen the data you wish to present, the next step is to select a presentation based on the type of data. Consider whether the data is quantitative or qualitative, whether you wish to display one or more variable and whether you wish to show trends over time or geographical variation. This will determine which type of data presentation can be used.

Types of Data Presentation

Tables

Tables can be useful for providing the reader with structured numeric information and can be used to present both categorical information and quantitative information, including frequency and cumulative frequency distributions, and associations between two or more variables using contingency tables.

Consider the purpose of the table. Reference tables provide information that the reader can look up and are often found in appendices. Demonstration tables present less information in a simple format that can be quickly understood by the reader, and are usually presented within the main text. Both types of tables should ideally fit onto one page to aid readability.

There are a few guidelines which can help you to produce high quality, easily understandable tables which convey your key messages:

- The orientation of information can affect understanding. People find it easier to make comparisons between information within a column than information within a row.
- The ordering can also impact the reader's understanding of the information within a table. If possible, present the rows in descending order for the most important column.
- Carefully consider the number of decimal points and use them consistently within and between tables. The minimum number of decimal points should be used whilst still accurately presenting the information. Too many decimal points can affect the readability and understanding of the table, and may imply the value is more accurate than it really is (especially for sample data).
- The rows and columns should be clearly labelled and include the units of measure.
- There should be no unnecessary information or formatting in the table—vertical column lines, for example, are rarely necessary within a table.

Charts

Charts are useful visual aids to support the reader to quickly understand the key messages from the data. There are many different types of charts available for use and the choice will depend primarily on the type of data that is being presented. We generally use charts for one or more of five main purposes:

- To compare data
- To show the distribution of data
- To show composition or part-to-whole relationships
- To show the relationships between variables
- To show trends over time

Key Principles in Data Presentation

There is considerable literature on how to present data; some of it comes from a design perspective, some from psychological research. Edward Tufte—one of the gurus of graphical presentation identifies what he calls "principles of graphical excellence". These include:

- Give the viewer the greatest number of ideas in the shortest time with the least ink in the smallest space. Presentations adhering to these principles tend to include small multiples (comparisons, and multivariate).

- Use clear, detailed and thorough labelling.
- Show data variation not design variation
- Maximise the amount of "data-ink". This is the element of a chart designed to show the data and allow its interpretation. This concords with the psychological principle in visualisation of salience—making the data the most important element of any display. Applying Tufte's principles means that "less is more"—often we add unnecessary colours, notation and lines which don't aid interpretation—Tufte calls these adornments "Chartjunk".

For more information see http://ieg.ifs.tuwien.ac.at/~gschwand/teaching/info-vis_ue_ws10/download/Principles%20of%20Graphical%20Excellence.pdf and we recommend reading Tufte's books.

Other commentators on data presentation include Stephen Few who has an excellent blog—Perceptual Edge (http://www.perceptualedge.com)—with step by step guides for a range of effective data displays including a one page guide to graph selection http://www.perceptualedge.com/articles/misc/Graph_Selection_Matrix.pdf.

Nature Methods run an excellent series of articles on scientific data display.

The graphic below shows some of the options for data display depending on the type of data and what you want to show.

Chart Suggestions—A Thought-Starter

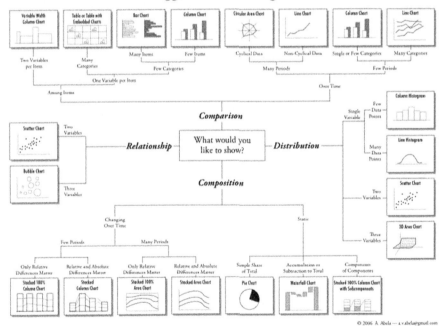

© 2006 A. Abela — a.v.abela@gmail.com

Qualitative (Categorical) Information: Composition Charts

There are a number of different chart types that can be used to present the frequency (or relative frequency) of data within each category.

Pie Charts

Pie charts present data in a circle which is divided into areas that are proportion to the frequency or relative frequency within each category. Each segment of the pie should be clearly labelled with the category and the frequency (or relative frequency).

Although commonly used to display categorical information, a disadvantage of pie charts is that people find it more difficult to estimate areas than lines. It is also difficult to compare the size of segments of the pie which are not next to each other.

Bar Chart

An alternative way to present categorical data is a bar chart. The categories are listed along the *x* axis and the frequency or relative frequency is on the *y* axis. The length of the bar is proportional to the frequency or relative frequency. It may be useful to label the actual frequency (or relative frequency) at the end of each bar, although this isn't necessary as, unlike pie charts, the *y* axis allows the reader to more easily estimate the frequency in each category.

If you wish to display another variable, you may wish to add further colour-coded bars to each category or consider using a stacked bar chart. If you choose to use either of these approaches, a legend must be used to clearly describe each variable. A line can be added to display an average or target frequency.

A bar chart must have gaps between each bars (unlike a histogram) to indicate that the categories on the *x* axis are not continuous.

Categorical Variables

Quantitative Information

Frequency or Relative Frequency of a Single Variable: Distribution Charts

Histogram

A histogram is used to show the frequency distribution of quantitative information. The data values are divided into intervals which are sometimes called "bins". The intervals are displayed on the *x* axis and the frequency or relative frequency of

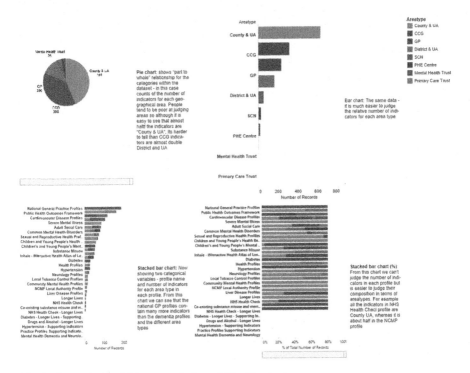

Fig. 1 Categorical variables—top single variable. *Pie chart*

values within each interval is displayed on the y axis. The height of each bar is proportional to the frequency (or relative frequency). Unlike bar charts, there are no gaps between each bar as the data intervals are continuous.

Histograms are useful to demonstrate the shape of the distribution and quickly tell us whether the data are distributed symmetrically or are positively or negatively skewed. They can also give us information on key measures such as the mean, median and mode. Error bars, such as confidence intervals, can be added to each histogram bar to give us further information about the variation of the data. Histograms do not allow us to read exact data values as the data is grouped into intervals and cannot be used to compare two sets of data.

Frequency Polygon (or Kernel Density Plots)

A frequency polygon is also used to show a frequency distribution. It is drawn by joining the midpoints of each histogram bar to make a smooth line and clearly demonstrates the shape of the distribution of data. An advantage of frequency polygons is that they can be used to compare two or more sets of data by drawing them on the same diagram.

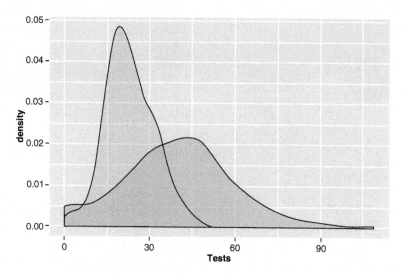

Fig. 2 Density plots comparing the distribution of CCG rates of two blood tests—PSA (*blue*) and ACR (*pink*) (colour figure online)

Box and Whisker Plot

Box and whisker plots are used to display the distribution of values of a quantitative variable and are constructed using the median, interquartile range, outliers, and the minimum and maximum values.

The box is drawn from the lower to the upper quartile and the length gives the interquartile range. The horizontal line in the middle of the box represents the median. The whiskers are then drawn to the maximum and minimum non-outlying values. Outlying values are displayed as individual points.

Box and whisker plots therefore display a wealth of information about the data including measures of central location (median), dispersion (range and interquartile range), outliers and whether the data is symmetrical or skewed. Two or more sets of data can be compared by presenting a box and whisker plot for each data set side by side. Like histograms, they do not allow us to read exact values (apart from the outlying points).

Other Kinds of Distributional Plots

Other kinds of plots used to show distributions include:

- Bee swarm plots (or distribution dot plots). These show all the data values as a scatter plot in binned in a similar way to histograms and give a clear sense of the shape of the distribution.
- Violin plots. These are kernel density plots which show the shape of this distribution as an outline. They can also contain a box plot which shows the centre of the distribution
- Bean plots. These show each data point as well as the outline of the distribution.

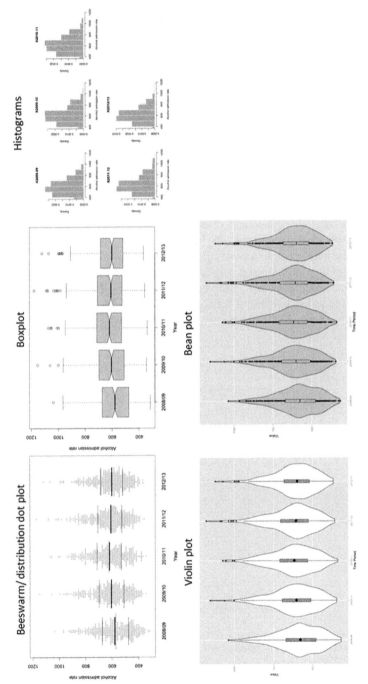

Fig. 3 Showing distributions—alcohol related admissions over time. Charts created in R using beeswarm package, ggplot2

Relationship Between Two Variables

Scatter Plots

Scatter plots are used to display the relationship between two continuous variables. One variable (usually the outcome variable) is displayed on the y axis, whilst the other variable (usually the exposure variable) is displayed on the x axis. Each individual value is then plotted as a data point. A trend line or line of best fit can then be added to aid interpretation and you may wish to display a measure of correlation (such as R^2) to describe the strength of the association.

Scatter plots provide a clear visual representation of the relationship between two variables and retain all of the data. They help us to assess whether there is an association between the variables, whether this association is positive or negative, whether it is linear or non-linear and whether the association is strong or weak (by observing the spread of points across the line). We can also see how large the sample size is by the number of data points that are plotted.

When interpreting scatter plots, it is important to remember that an association between two variables does not imply causation, and the Bradford Hill criteria should be used to assess whether it is likely that a change in the exposure variable causes the outcome variable to change.

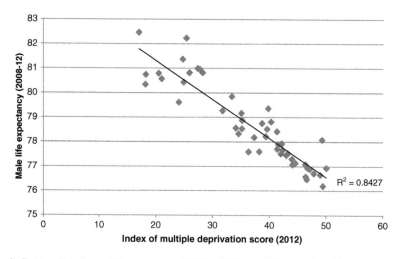

Fig. 4 Scatter plot of male life expectancy (2008—2012) at MSOA level and index of multiple deprivation score (2012) for all GP practices within an England Clinical Commissioning Group. Data source: PHE National General Practice Profiles (http://fingertips.phe.org.uk/)

Trends Over Time

Line Graphs

Changes over time of a quantitative variable can be displayed using a line graph in which time is displayed on the x axis and the variable is displayed on the y axis. More than one variable can be displayed on a line graph by adding lines; when this is done a legend must be displayed to clearly describe what each line represents.

You must ensure you have enough data points to display a meaningful trend over time. In addition, the scale on the y axis must be carefully selected in order to ensure that changes over time are not under- or overemphasised.

Maps

Maps can be a highly effective way of presenting health information to demonstrate geographical variation. The most commonly used type of map in health intelligence is the choropleth map. This is when graded differences in shading or colour are used to indicate the average value of a variable in a pre-defined area.

The first step in creating a choropleth map is to aggregate the data to your desired level; this may be, for example, super output area, ward or county. Mapping software can then be used to display the aggregated value for each area. It is often most visually effective and easily understandable to use different shadings of one colour. Symbols can be used to display other key geographical features such as the location of specific health services. Choropleth maps can also be displayed side by side to demonstrate whether there may be similar geographical variation observed in two or more variables.

Infographics

Infographics are an increasingly popular way to present a "story" using data and information. The Oxford Dictionary defines an infographic as "a visual representation of information or data, e.g. a chart or diagram". In practice, the term is usually used to display a wealth of data and information in one image using a variety of different types of visualisations and illustrations. They can be effectively used to clearly highlight key messages in a more accessible way than traditional formats such as text, tables and charts alone.

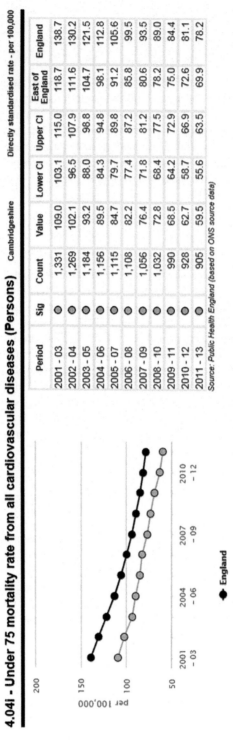

4.04i - Under 75 mortality rate from all cardiovascular diseases (Persons)

Period	Sig	Count	Value	Lower CI	Upper CI	East of England	England
2001 - 03	○	1,331	109.0	103.1	115.0	118.7	138.7
2002 - 04	○	1,269	102.1	96.5	107.9	111.6	130.2
2003 - 05	○	1,184	93.2	88.0	98.8	104.7	121.5
2004 - 06	○	1,156	89.5	84.3	94.8	98.1	112.8
2005 - 07	○	1,115	84.7	79.7	89.8	91.2	105.6
2006 - 08	○	1,108	82.2	77.4	87.2	85.8	99.5
2007 - 09	○	1,056	76.4	71.8	81.2	80.6	93.5
2008 - 10	○	1,032	72.8	68.4	77.5	78.2	89.0
2009 - 11	○	990	68.5	64.2	72.9	75.0	84.4
2010 - 12	○	928	62.7	58.7	66.9	72.6	81.1
2011 - 13	○	905	59.5	55.6	63.5	69.9	78.2

Cambridgeshire / Directly standardised rate - per 100,000

Source: Public Health England (based on ONS source data)

Fig. 5 Line graph and table showing premature mortality (under 75 years) from cardiovascular disease for Cambridgeshire and England, 2001-03 to 2010-12. Taken from PHE Public Health Outcomes Framework fingertips tool (http://fingertips.phe.org.uk/)

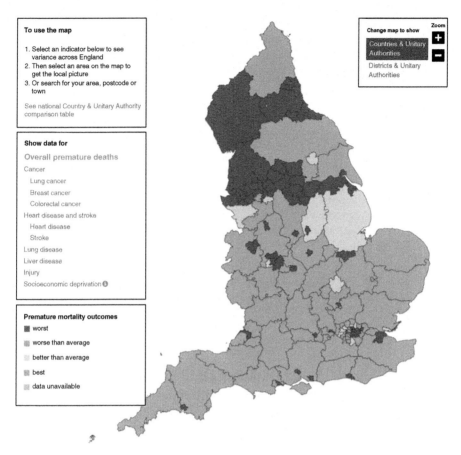

To use the map

1. Select an indicator below to see variance across England
2. Then select an area on the map to get the local picture
3. Or search for your area, postcode or town

See national Country & Unitary Authority comparison table

Show data for

Overall premature deaths
Cancer
  Lung cancer
  Breast cancer
  Colorectal cancer
Heart disease and stroke
  Heart disease
  Stroke
Lung disease
Liver disease
Injury
Socioeconomic deprivation ❶

Premature mortality outcomes
■ worst
▨ worse than average
☐ better than average
▨ best
▨ data unavailable

Change map to show Zoom
Countries & Unitary Authorities ➕
Districts & Unitary Authorities ➖

Fig. 6 Map of premature mortality (under 75 years) in England taken from the Public Health England Longer Lives tool (http://healthierlives.phe.org.uk)

Key Principles of Data Presentation

No matter what type of presentation you choose to use, there are some key principles which should be adhered to.

Key Principles
1. Tables and graphs should be self-explanatory—the reader should not have to refer to the text to understand them.
2. They should be clearly labelled, although not cluttered with unnecessary information.

3. Everything on the figure should add value—ink should not be wasted on either unnecessary information or formatting.
4. Do not use 3D or other special effects which can be misleading or make the presentation harder to understand.
5. The presentation should not be misleading—carefully consider the use of scales and use a jagged line to indicate that the axis does not start at zero. If you are presenting more than one chart alongside each other, use the same axis scales.
6. Put your most important data on the x and y axes, and use colours and shapes for the less important data.
7. Limit the number of colours and shapes used for clarity.
8. Use a legend to label colours and shapes clearly.
9. Consider the choice of font to make sure it is legible and present labels horizontally.
10. Check the presentation once finished—ask yourself whether it conveys your key messages, whether it is appropriate for the intended audience and whether it meets these key principles.

Worked Example: From Data to Insight Using Data Presentation—Example of Aortic Aneurysm Surgery (https://public.tableau.com/profile/musicwallaby31#!/vizhome/Chapter/Thedata)

1. *We showed the bubble plot earlier* (https://public.tableau.com/profile/musicwallaby31#!/vizhome/Chapter/Bubbleplot). *This was intended to show the variation in death rates between NHS trusts where the area of each bubble is proportional to the death rate. Psychological research shows that our visual perception of area is not as good as linear distance* (Cleveland and McGill 1987; Cleveland et al. 1982). *We can distinguish the length of bars or columns more accurately than the area of circles. For this reason bar charts are preferable for encoding multiple values to be compared than bubble charts (and stacked bar charts are better than Pie charts for "part-to-whole" relationships)* (*see* Ancker et al. 2006; Cleveland and McGill 1985).
2. *Bar charts should be presented ranked by value rather than alphabetically—we can then see the range of the data—who is at the bottom and the top, and sometimes learn from the shape of the distribution.* http://www.perceptualedge.com/articles/ie/the_right_graph.pdf   (https://public.tableau.com/profile/musicwallaby31#!/vizhome/Chapter/Rankedbar)

3. *We can improve things further by adding reference lines, e.g. the national average, to aid comparison with a benchmark.* (https://public.tableau.com/profile/musicwallaby31#!/vizhome/Chapter/Columnwithextrainf)

4. *Evidence based public health practice requires we have a measure of uncertainty on the estimates of mortality such as confidence intervals—if we reduce the bars to a point representing the value encoded by the bar we now have what is called a "caterpillar plot".* (https://public.tableau.com/profile/musicwallaby31#!/vizhome/Chapter/Caterpillar1)

5. *This chart nicely shows the variation and levels of uncertainty and (with some difficulty) we can tell outliers (areas which are statistically higher or lower than the national average) and tell that whether the high and low performers are different from one another.*

6. *Caterpillar plots and bar charts still suffer from the inherent weaknesses of ranking methods. Someone always has to be top and bottom of any set of comparative data and ranks are statistically unstable.*

7. *For this reason, new methods like funnel plots are now recommended for displaying performance data of this type* (Rakow et al. 2015; Spiegelhalter 2005). *They have several advantages over other methods of display:*

   (a) *They avoid ranking and take into account sample size or precision of estimates (in this case the mortality rate for Scarborough was based on a small number of cases)*

   (b) *They compare the actual distribution of mortality rates against the expected distribution so we can see how much of the variation between mortality rates is due to chance alone, and easily detect outliers ("special cause variation")*

   (c) *We can see if there is a volume outcome relationship*

   (d) *Clinicians are increasingly comfortable with this type of data presentation*

   (e) *There is recent empirical evidence that with minor modifications they can be presented to and be understood by the public*

   (f) *They can be used to partition variation into chance and non-chance and create colour schemes which can then be re-presented on maps or other charts—this approach is used in Longer Lives, for example* (http://healthier-lives.phe.org.uk).

   (g) *There are some downsides—they are complicated to draw in Excel—for this reason there are helpful templates for commonly used public health data that you can use to create them (or you can draw them in stats packages if you have the skill)—see* http://www.apho.org.uk/resource/item.aspx?RID=39445

   (h) *There is also a debate about correction for over-dispersion which is beyond the scope of this chapter.*

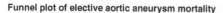

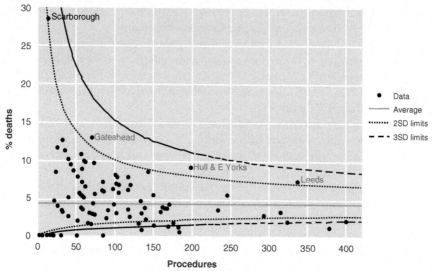

Funnel plot of elective aortic aneurysm mortality

Source: Guardian

8. *In this case the funnel plot shows:*

   (a) *The average mortality from elective aneurysm surgery is about 3.5 %*
   (b) *Most trusts lie within the funnel—they are indistinguishable from the national average*
   (c) *Although Scarborough has a high mortality rate this is based on small number of operations, but there are three other trusts who are potential outliers who undertake much higher volumes of surgery and these are where the attention should probably focus (although Scarborough probably did too few procedures to be viable).*
   (d) *Note that the this way of presenting the data treats all trust as part of a **system** with an average performance of 3.5 % and by and large this is the level most trusts perform at.*

Interactive Data Visualisation

Benefits of Interactivity

There is considerable interest in more interactive tools for charting and visualising data. There are a wide range of tools which can handle large numbers of indicators and large amounts of data which make it easier for users to understand and interpret the data, and save time. Interactivity means that data can be looked at it in meetings, shown on mobile devices and presented in novel ways for a range of audiences.

Examples (e.g. Fingertips, Gapminder)

Tools which come pre-populated with indicators include Fingertips (http://finger-tips.phe.org.uk) and Gapminder (http://www.gapminder.com). Gapminder makes use of animation in the form of a "Motion chart" (see below). Fingertips is a poweful tool for displaying a range of public health datasets in an interactive form making use of maps, heat maps, bar charts and funnel plots, trellis or panel charts and specially designed "small multiple" displays known as spine charts which plot multiple indicators for single areas compared with a range of benchmarks in a profile form.

Discussion Task
Exploring Gapminder. Load Gapminder into your browser (http://www.gap-minder.org/world). Select Zimbabwe from the country panel and press play (keep the Trails box checked).

- What happened to life expectancy in Zimbabwe in the 1990s? What happened to per capita income between 2001 and 2008.
- What explanations can you think of for these changes?
- What has happened since 2008?
- What might have caused this?

  Now select Russia and repeat the exercise

- What happened to life expectancy and per capita income in the 1990s

- What might explain this?

Doing It Yourself

Excel

By far the commonest tools used for creating charts and showing data are spread-sheet tools like Excel. They are hugely powerful and flexible and can create most types of chart people normally use such as histograms, line charts, bar and column charts and scatter plots. The latest version of excel includes the ability to draw spar-klines and bullet charts.

Some charts are more difficult to create like box plots and scatter plot matrices but there is a large online expert community which can provide help, and a range of excel add-ons and templates.

For example, to create funnel plots you can download templates from www.apho.org.uk and sites like Juice labs provide a range of templates for different types of chart presentation. http://labs.juiceanalytics.com/chartchooser/index.html

Stats Packages (Include R, Stata, SPSS, StatsDirect)

There are many stats packages available all of which have charting capability. Packages like R are free and are reputed to have some of the most flexible and best quality graphing capability supported by a large user community. There is quite a steep learning curve but its flexibility and power will mean that it will be increasingly used and taught. Packages like SPSS and Stata have more readymade graphics and many people learn the basics of one or other of these on public health courses.

Business Intelligence Tools

There are numerous tools designed to help you visualise data often called Exploratory Data Analysis or EDA tools. There is a good guide to evaluating these tools available at http://www.perceptualedge.com/articles/visual_business_intelligence/evaluating_visual_eda_tools.pdf. The best known are Tableau, Spotfire and Qlikview which vary in ease of use and cost. In the author's view Tableau public is one of the best and most flexible tools for rapid data exploration and evaluation. It has limited connectivity to data—only allowing links to text files and excel files, and a limitation of one million rows, but has enormous flexibility and power for creating visualisations and publishing them on the web and best of all its free!

We have used some examples throughout this chapter and recommend looking at this example relating toEbola to see how it can be used for public health monitoring and surveillance. http://healthintelligence.drupalgardens.com/content/tracking-ebola-virus-disease-outbreakwest-africa-2014.

This visualisation allows us to see how the Ebola outbreak spread, its lethality and progression and made a contribution to managing the outbreak.

Conclusion

Public health practice depends on data and clear and accurate presentation is a key skill. It is important not just to be able to present data but communicate results and impact clearly and be able to translate findings into action. We need to be able to say what data says, why it says it and what it means for policy and practice. In general less is more for clarity of presentation, avoiding information overload and storytelling. The sources of data for public health are increasing beyond traditional data collections into data from mobile phones to measure well-being and physical activity. The visualisation of data is a rapidly growing discipline in its own right with a growing evidence base, the development of powerful new tools to display and interact with data and the rapid growth of datasets both in variety and size and should form a part of the public health analytical armamentarium and curriculum.

References

Ancker, J. S., Senathirajah, Y., Kukafka, R., & Starren, J. B. (2006). Design features of graphs in health risk communication: A systematic review. *Journal of the American Medical Informatics Association, 13*(6), 608–618.

Cleveland, W. S., Harris, C. S., & McGill, R. (1982). Judgments of circle sizes on statistical maps. *Journal of the American Statistical Association, 77*(379), 541–547.

Cleveland, W. S., & McGill, R. (1985). Graphical perception and graphical methods for analyzing scientific data. *Science, 229*(4716), 828–833.

Cleveland, W. S., & McGill, R. (1987). Graphical perception: The visual decoding of quantitative information on graphical displays of data. *Journal of the Royal Statistical Society Series A (General), 150*(3), 192–229.

Rakow, T., Wright, R. J., Spiegelhalter, D. J., & Bull, C. (2015). The pros and cons of funnel plots as an aid to risk communication and patient decision making. *British Journal of Psychology, 106*, 327–348.

Spiegelhalter, D. J. (2005). Funnel plots for comparing institutional performance. *Statistics in Medicine, 24*(8), 1185–1202.

Recommended Reading

Cleveland, W. S. (1993). *Visualizing data*. Summit, NJ: Hobart Press.

Few, S. (2006). *Beautiful evidence: A journey through the mind of Edward Tufte. Mind*. Retrieved from http://www.b-eye-network.com/view/3226

Few, S. (2009). *Now you see it: Simple visualization techniques for quantitative analysis. Distribution*. Oakland, CA: Analytics Press.

Perceptual Edge. (2004). Visual business intelligence. Retrieved September 23, 2015, from www.perceptualedge.com.

Tufte, E. R. (1986). *Visual & statistical thinking: Displays of evidence for decision making*. Cheshire, CT: Graphics Press.

Tufte, E. R. (1997). *Visual explanations: Images and quantities, evidence and narrative*. Cheshire, CT: Graphics Press.

The Future Directions of Health Intelligence

Alison Hill and Julian Flowers

Abstract This chapter looks at the changing landscape of public health intelligence. It explores the concept of knowledge as an active social process, which adds value and achieves better health outcomes. Rapid developments in digital technology have opened horizons not envisaged 10 years ago. We look at the emergence of *big data* and its associated new discipline of *data science*, and consider the new data frontiers that will drive changes in health intelligence. We discuss the limits of traditional hypothesis testing and empirical research, and explore the emerging public health research paradigm. We look at the concept of knowledge management, and the global, national and local systems that are required for public health professionals to undertake their roles effectively and efficiently. Skills development goes hand in hand with these changes, and we discuss developments in health literacy, and the future public health knowledge workforce. The next decade will be one where the most significant developments will be in human systems and the human interface with technology, creating the cultural changes that will ensure delivery of the right knowledge to the right people at the right time.

After reading this chapter, you should be able to:

- Describe the nature of *big data,* the new data sources that are becoming available, and the challenges and opportunities that *big data* creates.
- Explain the emerging public health research paradigm, and the reasons why traditional empirical research is no longer appropriate for addressing complex public health interventions.
- Describe the concept of knowledge management, and the systems that are required to ensure that public health professionals can access the right knowledge at the right time.

A. Hill (✉)
Better Value Healthcare Ltd., Summertown Pavilion,18-24 Middle Way,
Oxford OX2 7LG, UK
e-mail: 4lison.hill@gmail.com

J. Flowers
Knowledge and Intelligence Service, Public Health England,
West Wing, Victoria House, Capital Park, Cambridge CB21 5XB, UK
e-mail: Julian.flowers@phe.gov.uk

© Springer International Publishing Switzerland 2016
K. Regmi, I. Gee (eds.), *Public Health Intelligence*,
DOI 10.1007/978-3-319-28326-5_12

- Identify the importance of health literacy in improving health outcomes and describe the contribution health intelligence and knowledge make to improving health literacy.
- Appreciate the blend of skills that the new public health intelligence workforce requires to take advantage of the changing nature of public health knowledge.
- Assess what will be different in 10 years time and determine the implications for your practice.

Introduction

Public health practice is based on knowledge. There is a long, strong and honourable tradition within the public health of the use of evidence and information going back to the nineteenth century. Epidemiology is the foundation of our speciality and is a core module of any public health curriculum. Partly because of its roots in the specialty of medicine the focus of evidence and data has tended to be biomedical and reductionist in its approach. But this book demonstrates that there is a sea change in the nature of the knowledge we are now using to inform public health policy and practice. This change brings both challenge and opportunity, which we review in this chapter.

Public health knowledge has three elements—research, routine data and experience. Each of these is, on its own, necessary but not sufficient. None stand alone, and bringing them together creates a whole that is greater than the sum of the parts. No policy and practice can be based on just one of these elements.

The word knowledge is not widely used within public health but is an essential all-encompassing term, and it is one that will be used increasingly in future. Definitions are important for creating common language and for bringing clarity and understanding, and this is a field that is fraught with terminological difficulties (Graham et al. 2006). Here we are using the term knowledge as the product of the component parts, that is the result of knowledge translation. Nonaka (1995) sees knowledge as information combined with human dynamism, implying that knowledge is an active social process, whereas information is passive.

This chapter looks to the future in the context of the changing landscape of health intelligence and knowledge. We don't know all that lies ahead, but here we assess emergent themes and consider how those might influence the future.

Future Sources of Data

Traditionally we have based public health practice on observation—collecting data about events or phenomena that have already happened and making inferences about observed variation or patterns in the data. We are familiar, for example, with John Snow's inferences about the patterns of cholera occurrence, which led him to conclude it was waterborne and to intervene to curtail the outbreak.

We mention this because the most significant recent developments in data in all fields is the emergence of the concept of *big data* and associated *data science,* which is the science of extracting insight and meaning from data of any kind for the purpose of driving change. In public health we are primarily concerned with changing behaviour, be it of citizens, practitioners, institutions or politicians; increasingly data is a powerful tool to assist us. If we are going to change behaviour with data we need to exploit relevant data from wherever it might come, breaking down some of the silos which exist (e.g. disease specific registration, disconnected surveillance systems), and link or "mash-up" disparate data sources. We will need to learn a new set of analytical, data management skills, and statistical techniques (e.g. machine learning, Bayesian approaches), develop new tools, and there is pressure to act fast, as the growth in potentially useful data is exponential, and methodology marches on apace.

Big data is characterised by 5 "V"s:

- **Volume**—data at large or massive scale (requiring new computing solutions to store and process). As the cost of storage has fallen the ability to scale up data is no longer a concern. This in turn has made the ability to store and process real time streams of data, and to "datify" everyday life much easier. If data can be stored it can be processed, and if it can be processed it can be analysed. Data at these volumes (gigabytes, terabytes and beyond) cannot be managed by the traditional spreadsheet approaches, and may exceed conventional database solutions.
- **Variety**—data of public health value is increasingly coming from different sources and in different forms. Increasingly data is *unstructured*—not conforming to any pre-defined schema (as opposed to health and care data which often follows strict schema). Examples of this include data from social media, health apps, news feeds and so on. There is considerable interest and research in early warning systems based on social media activity, for example.
- **Velocity**—as we discussed above, the speed at which data is available for processing is now real-time or near real-time for many things. In the health system however we are still often working with very out-of-date data, often years out-of-date, which lack credibility and utility, while we already have data collection systems which are capable of delivering more timely output.
- **Veracity**—just because data is "big" doesn't mean it is accurate or true, or of sufficient quality to draw valid inferences. There is potential for biases (particularly selection bias), confounding and poor data quality, which limit the value of any analysis. It should also be noted that much analysis of *big data* generates associations that may be spurious, and from which we can only generate hypotheses.
- **Value**—if we are going to invest heavily in *big data* infrastructure, skills and time into big data we need to demonstrate return on that investment in terms of change, improvement and so on. We therefore need to avoid "fishing exercises" and try and focus on high value questions where we need new insight, and we need to build in evaluation at the start.

Public health practitioners are well placed to use big data judiciously. Their strong analytical background and training in critical appraisal and epidemiology will help avoid "big data hubris" which is a phrase reflecting the belief that *big data* can substitute for conventional approaches (Lazer et al. 2014).

There are probably five "data frontiers" which will drive change in health intelligence over the next 10 years.

1. **Primary care data.** In the UK we are fortunate to have increasing availability of primary care data, from GP clinical systems. The potential of primary care data in research is well demonstrated and there is increasing recognition of their public health value in support of new models of population-based healthcare and preventive services. As an example of public health potential, GPs, through the Quality and Outcome Framework (QOF) system, have had financial incentives to record the smoking status of their practice populations. We know that around 86 % of the over-15 population has had their smoking status recorded in the previous 2 years.[1] However QOF has never published the results of smoking status (i.e. how many people are recorded as current smokers). It has, however, now become possible to calculate smoking prevalence from combining QOF indicators (Honeyford et al. 2014). From these data we have an estimate of smoking prevalence of 19.1 % for 2013/2014 based on a sample size of many millions, and we can estimate prevalence for every general practice, clinical commissioning group, and local authority, with these data (Fig. 1). Although the current basis for prevalence estimation is the Integrated Household Survey, GP data gives the potential for monitoring smoking, and other risk factors, based on much larger samples, that is cheaper, more timely and more granular (Langley et al. 2011).

2. **Linked data.** Data linkage is not new and has delivered important insights over the past 30 years (Roberts and Goldacre 2003). It is very much at the heart of thinking about healthcare data for the next few years. It is recognised that sharing data across different services is essential for integrated care, care delivery, outcomes development and research. Notwithstanding the methodological and information governance challenges (see below), considerable investment is being made to link healthcare data more systematically and robustly, for example, *care. data* and the Farr Institute.

3. **Social network and other unstructured data.** There are a number of potential sources of data, of which Twitter and outputs of web searching are the most researched. Google Flu trends is the best known. It has been claimed that analysing web-based searches for flu and related search term has high predictive value for flu outbreaks and epidemics, and reacts more quickly than conventional flu surveillance systems. Recent evidence however suggests that the Google flu service has considerably overestimated the size and scale of US flu outbreaks and that big data approaches still need to be treated with caution and need evaluation (Lazer et al. 2014). Similar methods have been applied to other diseases such as Dengue Fever (Gluskin et al. 2014) and TB (Zhou et al. 2011). Twitter feeds are being evaluated for their public health potential. Research has shown how

---

[1] http://bit.ly/1MxNjX0 from http://fingertips.phe.org.uk/profile/general-practice/

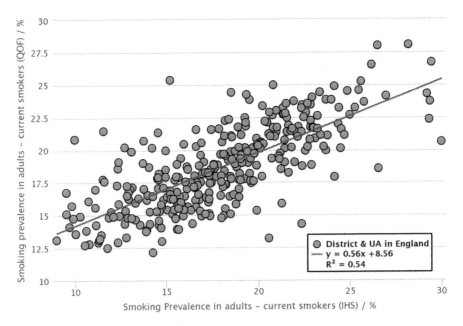

Fig. 1 Correlation between IHS and QOF based estimates of adults smoking for Local Authority populations in England. *Source*: Local Tobacco Profiles for England; analysis by authors; accessed August 2015

analysis of Twitter can generate descriptive epidemiological data for diseases which correlates well with conventional estimates, so there seems to be considerable potential (Paul et al. 2011).

4. **Mobile and app data and remote sensing.** Another future source of data will be from health apps, mobile phone networks and remote sensors such as fitness wearables, medical devices (e.g. blood pressure or vital signs monitors) and "the Internet of things". Already Apple is making anonymised data from the Apple Watch available (https://www.apple.com/uk/researchkit/). The sensors in mobile phones can monitor physical activity in real time as well as through GPS, and combine this with location information. This method of estimating physical activity for population monitoring will probably replace the crude self-reported, expensive monitoring data we currently get through surveys (taking into account the downsides of "big data" and biases inherent in this type of monitoring). It is likely that ever more sophisticated sensors will become available, capable of more powerful monitoring. This could provide real-time data on large cohorts of people, which might allow us to develop predictive tools to guide individual tailored lifestyle advice, "personalised public health" and evaluate population-based interventions. Added to this, apps are available which allow self-reporting of well-being and this can all be combined to help us link well-being, lifestyles and risk factors in ways currently impossible.

5. **Data science.** None of this will be possible without building the analytical skills of the public health workforce, and developing a strong translation function. Making sense of all this data, turning into actionable outputs and communicating it clearly will be challenging and require further research into translation—preferably directly built into data collection and publication systems. There is also a need to break down data silos which prevent information sharing and new insight being generated from putting data from multiple sources along side one another and using new techniques to combined these datasets to make best use of what we know (Thompson et al. 2009).

Information Governance

At the same time as we are making more data accessible through the open data and transparency agenda, information governance barriers are restricting what we can do with the data and preventing vital knowledge being generated through linkage. There is no doubt that as more data is accessible, the risks to privacy grow, and some believe that it is not possible to completely protect everyone's data such that there is no risk to re-identification. This is a significant force pulling in the opposite direction to openness and wide publication.

In England this schism has been most keenly felt in the *care.data* debate. *Care. data* is a scheme designed to link together primary and secondary care data on a large scale for a wide range of purposes. The data required linkage at the patient level and therefore the use of patient identifiers. Because of the scale it would not be possible to obtain explicit patient consent for the data from general practices (for which GPs are data controllers) to be shared with Health and Social Care Information Centre (HSCIC), who control the secondary care data, in order for the HSCIC to do the linkage.

After much consultation, NHS England, commissioners of the project, agreed to provide "fair processing" information to every household as required by the Data Protection and the Information Commissioner's Office. This exercise surfaced a wide range of issues, stirred up the privacy lobby and called into question the uses of patient data leading to a "deficit of public trust" [real or perceived]. It sent the HSCIC, who under the Health and Social Care Act (HM Government 2012) have the legal mandate to collect and collate the data, into a period of introspection and review, which has prevented data sharing for commissioning, research and public health being shared and used. Public confidence may have been irreparably damaged.

For public health purposes, Public Health England has responsibility for ensuring the legal basis for data sharing and is working actively to navigate through the turbulent waters that constitute information governance.

We can only hope that we can emerge from the current situation with more clarity, appropriate permissiveness, and the ability to make best use of the data we have for public good.

Evidence from Research

Public health evidence comes from a variety of sources, published or unpublished empirical research, theory, narrative, experience, data and tacit knowledge. With its biomedical roots, there has been a general acceptance that evidence must reach a high level of quality and robustness to be of sufficient use to inform policy and practice. Public health research, with good reason, adopted the accepted hierarchy of evidence from the evidence-based practice movement (Guyatt et al. 1995). Controlled trials still have a major role to play where interventions are relatively simple and linear, but the world of public health is increasingly complex and messy. Many public health interventions are non-linear, multifaceted, and whole system, with less focus on targeted individual behaviour change, and more on other upstream contemporaneous environmental, societal and economic changes. Traditional technology appraisal is mainly around research at an individual level and is not a good fit with public health interventions (Fischer et al. 2013). There are parallels here with Rose's prevention paradox (Rose, 1981). Programmes targeted at individuals tend to be for a small number of high risk people and attract research funding, whereas there is a dearth of research into those interventions that may only have a small impact at an individual level but a large impact at a population level (shifting the whole curve). This means that the traditional views both of research and of the implementation of research evidence require new approaches. A new paradigm is therefore emerging.

Firstly public health evidence is increasingly coming from evaluation of large-scale programmes and natural experiments (Craig et al. 2012) rather than interventional research at individual level. Take, for example, interventions to increase cycling and walking within communities. Two systematic reviews (Ogilvie et al. 2007; Yang et al. 2010) have assessed interventions targeted at individuals to increase walking and cycling. The evidence from these systematic reviews was not definitive. This is because the literature is dominated by studies of individually targeted interventions to address behaviour change. Focusing purely on individual interventions does not take into account wider environmental, fiscal, social and cultural factors, and the research therefore addresses one small element in a wide set of influences. The narrowness of the reviews does not mean that individually targeted interventions are not effective, rather it means that the available research is too skewed towards particular kinds of invention to be able to answer the question of effectiveness at system level. For cycling and walking better evidence is coming from cluster randomised trials (Higgins et al. 2008), natural experiments, and evaluations of large population based programmes that integrate transport and health evaluative approaches (Ogilvie et al. 2011; Sloman et al. 2009).

Secondly as randomised trials of public health interventions do not result in definitive outcomes a proposition is emerging that public health policy and practice should be influenced by decision theory based on theoretic assumptions, and empirical and experiential evidence, including costs (Threlfall et al. 2015). This approach uses Bayesian techniques requiring more upstream systems thinking, identifying all the levers, testing of options, and weighing the evidence across options.

For example, looking at obesity, much of the research has been on individual or group level responses such as bariatric surgery and weight management interventions. The randomised controlled trial evidence is that bariatric surgery is an effective and cost-effective intervention (Chang et al. 2014; Picot et al. 2009). However surgery is offered to a tiny proportion of the obese population and would be unaffordable if offered to all who might benefit. While modelling shows that a sugar drink tax could have an impact across a whole population (Briggs et al. 2013), there is no empirical evidence to support the introduction of such a tax. Furthermore it is likely to be part of a range of policies being introduced to tackle obesity, which makes it difficult, if not impossible, to test the specific impact of single interventions within the overall framework. Using a decision-theoretic approach, introduction of a sugar tax would use assumptions about impacts drawn from theory, empirical evidence drawn from observation and natural experiments, and experience, using transparent assumptions that are challengeable, to assess the case for the introduction of such a tax.

Thirdly and linked to both of the previous two developments, public health research must incorporate community and citizen knowledge, lived experience and insights, into the evidence base, to create an understanding of how communities use services and respond to interventions, and what the impacts of, and impacts on, health inequalities are. Without this interventions based on research can be meaningless and irrelevant when implemented in real-world situations. The public health research community must work in partnership with communities to understand their needs and experience to inform research, particularly when it impacts on health inequalities. New academic-community collaborations, such as community-campus partnerships, are emerging (South et al. 2014), which are modelling this approach. Co-creation between researchers and communities is fundamental to the future of public health research.

Over the next few years therefore we will see growing recognition of the limits of hypothesis testing research looking at individual behaviour change. Research interest will shift to a broader range of evidence taken from observations of, and involvement with, communities and populations, and decisions will draw much more on option testing using decision theory. The most important interventions are societal, and research techniques and focus need to shift in recognition of that.

Knowledge Management

Managing knowledge is a key public health responsibility for the twenty-first century. Gray (2005) graphically compares the management of knowledge to that of water, which was a key public health responsibility of the nineteenth century. The public and professionals need access to clean, clear knowledge available on tap when and where it is needed. With the coming of the digital age, we are bombarded and overloaded with information, and knowledge management is the way we address this overload and get what we need on tap. The goal of knowledge management is to "deliver the right information to the right person and place at the right time" (Association of State and Territorial Health Officials 2005), and is a prerequisite for managing successful public health programmes.

Knowledge management developed as a scientific discipline in its own right in the early 1990s, spearheaded by Nonaka and Takeuchi (Nonaka 1995). It was seen as giving companies competitive advantage, and became mainstream at the start of this century. The twenty-first century is the era of knowledge, coined the "knowledge society" by Drucker, where knowledge is the key resource, of equivalent importance to financial and human resources, knowledge workers being the main workforce (Drucker 2001). Digital technology and the evolution of the internet have been the engines behind the growth of knowledge management as a discipline. However, the health and public health sector have been slow to take up knowledge management systematically, being subjected to constant change due to political influence, and failing to invest (Kothari et al. 2011) .

This section takes a very high level overview of what knowledge management in public health requires, with a focus on technical knowledge required for public health action. Public health knowledge management is a highly complex networked system, requiring capture, organisation, translation, communication and use, based on common standards, at a global, national and local level. There are many different models of knowledge management in the literature (Kothari et al. 2011), but for public health the NHS National Library for Health identified three integrated components, technology, processes and people (NHS National Library for Health 2005), with Dubois and Wilkerson adding content and culture as two further essential components (Dubois and Wilkinson 2008). We look at each of these below.

1. **Content.** The creation of a global system for capturing research in databases such as MEDLINE® has been at the heart of public health knowledge (and other health and social sciences). The cataloguing and categorising of research papers and storage in databases using internationally agreed taxonomies and metadata standards is now taken for granted, building on a tradition that goes back to the nineteenth century.

   Systematic reviews exemplify pure filtered knowledge. The Campbell Library (http://www.campbellcollaboration.org) and the Cochrane Library (http://www.cochranelibrary.com) provide high quality reviews, and are examples of knowledge synthesis within a global system. Retrieval is the first filter, which is a systematic process of identification of relevant articles through expert searching using the appropriate search terms. Critical appraisal sifts the good from the poor and irrelevant, or worse, wrong and dangerous. Further purification is undertaken to ensure that diverse users can read the reviews. For instance, many Cochrane reviews have a plain language summary, which is written so that it is accessible to lay people.

   Whereas knowledge from research is managed at a global level, knowledge from routine statistics and surveys is held at a national level. For example, the four UK countries have national holdings of population statistics, hospital episode statistics, cancer registries, health survey data, and a vast array other data that inform wider determinants of health. Much knowledge translation is undertaken at national level, with the creation of tailored products, synthesising data and evidence into resources meaningful for different audiences.

At a local level the global and national knowledge resources are brought together within a local context, using knowledge derived from local communities. Knowledge translation is a key function of public health organisations and is the process of bringing together evidence, data, and community and professional experience in ways that make knowledge accessible and useable by the target user, whether the public, professionals within the public health system, and other decision-makers.

2. **Processes.** These are activities and initiatives that help facilitate knowledge management along the whole knowledge pipeline. They need to be designed around the knowledge requirements arising from an organisation's strategy. Processes need to be focused around how the organisation operates, and specifically around how knowledge is created, translated, used and shared.

3. **Technology.** Knowledge resources and products are all held in digital form, and need to be stored and catalogued in a way that the end user can retrieve them. It is the process by which users access clear clean knowledge at the time they want it, in the form they want it. There is an array of different tools and techniques available to knowledge managers, and web-based tools and websites, which allow for personalisation, using targeted, approaches with alerts and prompts. Social media is increasingly used in this way.

4. **People.** There are many players in public health knowledge management. These are information scientists doing the resource management, cataloguing, filtering, researchers doing appraisals, analysts doing the data analysis, public health professionals and science writers undertaking the knowledge translation and communication, and information technologists building and maintaining the many databases and digital tools to manage the resources. Within every organisation someone needs to be responsible for knowledge, and Public Health England has led the way through the creation of the post of Chief Knowledge Officer to oversee the generation, synthesis, translation and distribution of knowledge to the public health system across England.

5. **Culture.** All public health organisations need to generate a culture that values knowledge and sees it as a resource to share and build on (Dubois and Wilkinson 2008). This is going to be the greatest challenge of the next decade, to capture the tacit knowledge within organisations and communities, and make it explicit (Collins 2010), and to share and exchange knowledge in all its forms across the public health workforce. Only this way will we achieve the best outcomes for communities.

Health Literacy

The World Health Organization defines health literacy as "the personal characteristics and social resources needed for individuals and communities to access, understand, appraise and use information and services to make decisions about health" (Dodson et al. 2015).

Although not a major focus in this book we include a section on it here, as it is fundamental to improving health and reducing health inequalities, and is based on public health evidence and intelligence that is the heart of this book. An essential step in the knowledge pathway is knowledge translation to make evidence and intelligence accessible and interpretable by end users, and it is hard to argue that the most critically important end user is the citizen, who makes health and health care choices on the basis of that evidence and intelligence. Like health professionals, citizens need the skills to make use of knowledge to enhance health promoting behaviour, make better use of health services and preventive health services, and reduce waste in healthcare through better adherence to medication and self-care, all with the ultimate aim of improving health outcomes.

Low health literacy is associated with poorer longer term outcomes (Bostock and Steptoe 2012). Access to, and use of, evidence and intelligence show strong socio-demographic differential, contributing to the health inequalities differential experienced by people in lower socio-demographic groups, people with learning disabilities, or ethnic minorities with English as a second language. Such groups have knowledge and skills deficits that impact negatively on health improving behaviours, and in access to and use of health care (Greenhalgh 2015).

Health literacy is a complex concept that has emerged from two traditions, clinical medicine and health promotion (Nutbeam 2008). Two systematic reviews have helped to develop and extend the understanding of health literacy into a wider public health context, drawing on these traditions, while recognising that there is still debate on its measurement, the impacts of low health literacy, and the implications for action (Sorensen et al. 2012; Haun et al. 2014).

Nutbeam (2000) describes three types of health literacy, functional, interactive and critical. Functional is the basic literacy and numeracy skills to be able to understand and act on health information however presented. Interactive health literacy is about people having the confidence to discuss their health issues with professionals, to promote shared decision-making. Critical health literacy is about people taking control over wider health determinants. Evidence and intelligence informs all three types.

Producers of health information, in whatever medium, have a responsibility to ensure the quality of content and the style of communication is appropriate to the user. The Information Standard in England is a certification programme for organisations producing evidence-based health and care information for the public. Those organisations achieving The Information Standard have been accredited on the basis of producing information that is clear, accurate, balanced, evidence-based and up-to-date.

As the understanding of its impacts grows, there is an increasing recognition of the need to improve health literacy (Rowlands et al. 2014). This will require coordinated system-wide multifaceted approaches, involving the public and many players in policy, public health, healthcare, the media and researchers. Improving knowledge and skills of individuals and communities and their understanding of the concepts of health and its underpinning research is a core objective.

However this is only one part of the system. Health professionals and health communicators also have a responsibility to communicate in ways that are sensitive to the needs of the end user. Health professionals use face-to-face consultations to communicate essential health messages. They need to know how to communicate to widely diverse patients and clients. Producers of health information need to ensure that it meets accepted standards such as that of The Information Standard. No information resource should be designed without input from users. The aim of any health literacy programme is that communications are under the control of users, or if a product, are co-produced. We need the "development of a health-literate health system accessible to all, and empowered, health-literate patients …". (Rowlands et al. 2014).

The Future Workforce

Public health is a knowledge business, and the form that knowledge takes is becoming increasingly complex and heterogeneous. People working within the field search for, collect, analyse, appraise, interpret and communicate information about public health. This requires an increasing range and blend of analytic, critical and interpretive skills. In the UK the skills and knowledge competences have been set out in the Faculty of Public Health's specialty training guide curriculum (Faculty of Public Health 2010) and in the UK Public Health Skills and Knowledge Framework (PHORCAST 2013), but the way they have been articulated creates a distinct separation of the skills of finding and appraising evidence, and handling data and information, and focuses insufficiently on knowledge translation.

Increasingly, as this book and this chapter have shown, the public health intelligence workforce is having to work with more diverse sets of data and evidence sources, understand their strengths and weaknesses, integrate and interpret these complex inputs, and then translate and communicate that knowledge as meaningful outputs for a range of lay and professional audiences. To help them with these highly skilled and difficult tasks, health intelligence practitioners are using sophisticated tools and statistical and modelling techniques. But to create products, which are going to persuade and influence those different users, and win their hearts and minds, requires an understanding of the context and the audience, so this workforce needs cultural, sociological and psychological skills as well.

This means that the future practitioner will be moving beyond traditional epidemiological thinking and approaches, using novel data sources, and relying on evidence that is more experiential, and less robust than classic empirical research. In addition they need to understand how knowledge is absorbed and acted on by users, so have an understanding of the behavioural sciences.

Currently training is mainly on the job within local public health teams or national public health entities. There are no specific masters degrees in public health intelligence, and only a few dedicated training programmes. There are some professional bodies, such as health statistics user group of the Royal Statistical Society, that support current practitioners in upskilling and updating. The Skills and

Knowledge Framework has helped to codify the competencies and skills but as mentioned above it does not integrate the knowledge strands, and knowledge and skills requirements are now for integration and communication. There is a compelling and urgent need to rethink the training and development of this particular workforce to support them in taking up the extraordinary opportunities that are emerging within the field of public health knowledge.

...and in 10 Years Time

The staggering developments in digital technology would for most of us have been impossible to imagine 10 years ago. Mobiles were mainly used for phoning, until the first iPhone was introduced in 2007. Text messaging was still less popular than phoning. Twitter was invented in 2006. Superfast broadband was still not available in homes (it was introduced around 2010). Fast mobile broadband technology is still not universal. Interactive computer graphics have developed rapidly with new ways of presenting data. The availability of huge Cloud storage is transforming the way we interface with and access resources. You can no doubt add much more to that list.

It is therefore very difficult to predict what our world will be like 10 years ahead. Gibson[2] is reported as saying "The future is already here—it's just not very evenly distributed". At best in this forward look we have observed what is happening now and have extrapolated that, as that is all we are able to see.

In 2014 CNN invited Sir Tim Berners-Lee to share his thoughts on the future of the internet.[3] He was quoted as saying "Devices are getting cheaper and Internet access is slowly becoming universal, but how we use it is broken and needs to change". He set out the following developments as priorities for the future.

- Information needs to be regulated and controlled, especially our health data.
- Business will need to practice greater transparency.
- Banks need to practice better security.
- Pixels will get smaller.
- Public data is important and we will have more access to it.
- There will be a need for an Internet bill of rights to protect users.

You can see that apart from smaller pixels Berners-Lee's predictions are about ways of working, processes and regulation. This holds true for the future of public health intelligence and knowledge. Our prediction is that the accelerated changes in digital technology will start slowing and that for public health practice the next decade will be one where the major developments are in human skills, human systems and human interfaces with technology. We also have to rebuild the trust of the public that health data is safe in our hands. If we achieve these we will become truly effective as a public health knowledge workforce.

---

[2] https://en.wikiquote.org/wiki/William_Gibson

[3] http://edition.cnn.com/2014/12/23/business/tim-berners-lee-future-insights/

Acknowledgement We would like to thank Anne Brice, Prof. Harry Rutter and Prof. Sir Muir
Gray for their advice in preparing this chapter.

References

Association of State and Territorial Health Officials. (2005). *Knowledge management for public
health professionals.* Washington DC: ASTHO.

Bostock, S., & Steptoe, A. (2012). Association between low functional health literacy and mortality in older adults: Longitudinal cohort study. *British Medical Journal, 344*, e1602. doi:10.1136/
bmj.e1602.

Briggs, A. D., Mytton, O. T., Madden, D., O'Shea, D., Rayner, M., et al. (2013). The potential
impact on obesity of a 10% tax on sugar-sweetened beverages in Ireland, an effect assessment
modelling study. *BMC Public Health, 13*, 860. doi:10.1186/1471-2458-13-860.

Chang, S. H., Stoll, C. R., Song, J., Varela, J. E., Eagon, C. J., et al. (2014). The effectiveness
and risks of bariatric surgery: An updated systematic review and meta-analysis, 2003-2012.
Journal of American Medical Association Surgery, 149(3), 275–287. doi:10.1001/
jamasurg.2013.3654.

Collins, H. (2010). *Tacit and explicit knowledge.* Chicago: University of Chicago Press.

Craig, P., Cooper, C., Gunnell, D., Haw, S., Lawson, K., Macintyre, S., et al. (2012). Using natural
experiments to evaluate population health interventions: New Medical Research Council guidance. *Journal of Epidemiology and Community Health, 66*(12), 1182–1186. doi:10.1136/
jech-2011-200375.

Dodson, S., Good, S., & Osborne, R. H. (2015). *Health literacy toolkit for low- and middle-income
countries: A series of information sheets to empower communities and strengthen health systems.* New Delhi: World Health Organization.

Drucker, P. F. (2001). The next society. *The Economist, 8246*, 3–22.

Dubois, N., & Wilkinson, T. (2008). *Knowledge management: Backforund paper for the development of a knowledge management strategy for public health in Canada.* Hamilton, Canada:
National Collaborating Centre for Methods and Tools.

Faculty of Public Health. (2010). *Public health specialty training curriculum.* London: FPH.

Fischer, A. J., Threlfall, A., Meah, S., Cookson, R., Rutter, H., et al. (2013). The appraisal of public
health interventions: An overview. *Journal of Public Health, 35*(4), 488–494. doi:10.1093/
pubmed/fdt076.

Gluskin, R. T., Johansson, M. A., Santillana, M., & Brownstein, J. S. (2014). Evaluation of
Internet-Based Dengue Query Data: Google Dengue Trends. *PLoS Neglected Tropical
Diseases., 8*(2), e2713. doi:10.1371/journal.pntd.0002713.

Graham, I. D., Logan, J., Harrison, M. B., Straus, S. E., Tetroe, J., et al. (2006). Lost in knowledge
translation: Time for a map? *Journal of Continuing Education in the Health Professions, 26*(1),
13–24. doi:10.1002/chp.47

Gray, J. A. (2005). *A national public health knowledge service* (Vol. 6). London: Faculty of Public
Health, ph.com.

Greenhalgh, T. (2015). Health literacy: Towards system level solutions. *British Medical Journal,
350*, h1026. doi:10.1136/bmj.h1026.

Guyatt, G. H., Sackett, D. L., Sinclair, J. C., Hayward, R., Cook, D. J., et al. (1995). Users' guides
to the medical literature. *IX. A method for grading health care recommendations. Journal of the
American Medical Association, 274*, 1800–1804.

Haun, J. N., Valerio, M. A., McCormack, L. A., Sorensen, K., & Paasche-Orlow, M. K. (2014).
Health literacy measurement: An inventory and descriptive summary of 51 instruments. *Journal
of Health Communication, 19*(Suppl 2), 302–333. doi:10.1080/10810730.2014.936571.

Higgins, J. P. T., Deeks, J. J., & Altman, D. G. (2008). *Chapter 16: Special topics in statistics.
Cochrane Handbook for Systematic Reviews of Interventions.* Version 5.0.1 [updated September
2008]. The Cochrane Collaboration.

HM Government. (2012). *Health and Social Care Act 2012*. Norwich, England: HMG.

Honeyford, K., Baker, R., Bankart, M. J. G., & Jones, D. R. (2014). Estimating smoking prevalence in general practice using data from the Quality and Outcomes Framework (QOF). *British Medical Journal, 4*(7), e005217. doi:10.1136/bmjopen-2014-005217.

Kothari, A., Hovanec, N., Hastie, R., & Sibbald, S. (2011). Lessons from the business sector for successful knowledge management in health care: A systematic review. *BMC Health Services Research, 11*(1), 173–183. doi:10.1186/1472-6963-11-173.

Langley, T. E., Szatkowski, L. C., Wythe, S., & Lewis, S. A. (2011). Can primary care data be used to monitor regional smoking prevalence? An analysis of The Health Improvement Network primary care data. *BMC Public Health. 11*, 773. doi:10.1186/1471-2458-11-773.

Lazer, D., Kennedy, R., King, G., & Vespignani, A. (2014). The parable of Google Flu: Traps in Big Data analysis. *Science, 343*(6167), 1203–1205.

NHS National Library for Health. (2005). *ABC of Knowledge Management*. London: NHS.

Nonaka, I. T. H. (1995). *The knowledge-creating company*. How Japanese Companies Create the Dynamics of Innovation. London: Oxford University Press.

Nutbeam, D. (2000). Health literacy as a public health goal: A challenge for contemporary health education and communication strategies into the 21st century. *Health Promotion International, 15*(3), 259-267. doi:10.1093/heapro/15.3.259.

Nutbeam, D. (2008). The evolving concept of health literacy. *Social Science & Medicine, 67*(12):2072–2078. doi:10.1016/j.socscimed.2008.09.050.

Ogilvie, D., Bull, F., Powell, J., Cooper, A., Brand, C., et al. (2011). An applied ecological framework for evaluating infrastructure to promote walking and cycling: The iConnect study. *American Journal of Public Health*, 101, 473–481. doi:10.2105/AJPH.2010.198002.

Ogilvie, D., Foster, C. E., Rothnie, H., Cavill, N., Hamilton, V., Fitzsimons, C. F., & Mutrie, N. (2007). Interventions to promote walking: Systematic review. *British Medical Journal, 334*(7605), 1204. doi:10.1136/bmj.39198.722720.BE.

Paul, M. J., & Dredze, M.(2011). *You are what you tweet: Analyzing twitter for public health*. In: Proceedings of the Fifth International AAAI Conference on Weblogs and Social Media, 2011. pp. 265–272. doi:http://doi.org/10.1.1.224.9974.

Picot, J., Jones, J., Colquitt, J. L., Gospodarevskaya, E., Loveman, E., Baxter, L., et al. (2009). The clinical effectiveness and cost-effectiveness of bariatric (weight loss) surgery for obesity: A systematic review and economic evaluation. Health Technology Assessment, 13(41), 1–190, 215–357, iii–iv. doi:10.3310/hta13410.

PHORCAST. (2013). *UK public health skills and knowledge framework*. London: PHORCAST.

Roberts, S. E., & Goldacre, M. J. (2003). Case fatality rates after admission to hospital with stroke: Linked database study. *British Medical Journal, 326*, 1468–5833.

Rose, G. (1981). Strategy of prevention: Lessons from cardiovascular disease. *British Medical Journal, 282*, 1847–1851.

Rowlands, G., Protheroe, J., Price, H., Gann, B., & Rafi, I. (2014). *Health literacy. report from an RCGP-led health literacy workshop*. London: Royal College of General Practitioners.

Sloman, L., Cavill, N., Cope, A., Muller, L., & Kennedy, A. (2009). *Report for Department for Transport and Cycling England*. London: Department for Transport and Cycling. Analysis and synthesis of evidence on the effects of investment in six Cycling Demonstration Towns.

Sorensen, K., Van den Broucke, S., Fullam, J., Doyle, G., Pelikan, J., Slonska, Z., Brand, H., & European, C. H. L. P. (2012). Health literacy and public health: A systematic review and integration of definitions and models. *BMC Public Health, 12*(1), 80.

South, J., White, J., & Gamsu, M. (2014). *Putting 'the public' back into public health. Post conference briefing*. In: Putting 'the public' back into public health. A national conference on building the voice of citizens into public health evidence. Leeds, UK: Leeds Beckett University.

Thompson, S., Spiegelhalter, D., RM, T., & Flowers, J. R. (2009). *Estimating smoking prevalence in small areas by pooling data from multiple sources*. Paper presented at the Faculty of Public Health Annual Conference, Scarborough.

Threlfall, A., Meah, S., Fischer, A., Cookson, R., Rutter, H., & Kelly, M. (2015). The appraisal of public health interventions: The use of theory. *Journal of Public Health, 37*(1), 166–171.

Yang, L., Sahlqvist, S., McMinn, A., Griffin, S. J., & Ogilvie, D. (2010). Interventions to promote cycling: Systematic review. *British Medical Journal, 341*(7778), 870–870. doi:10.1136/bmj. c5293.

Zhou, X., Ye, J., & Feng, Y. (2011). Tuberculosis surveillance by analyzing Google trends. *Transactions on Biomedical Engineering, 58*(8), 2247–2254.

Recommended Reading

Sim, F., & Wright, J. (2015). *Working in public health: An introduction to careers in public health.* London: Routledge.

World Health Organisation. (2014). *Providing health intelligence to meet local needs: A practical guide to serving local and urban communities through public health observatories.* Geneva: WHO.

Index

© Springer International Publishing Switzerland 2016
K. Regmi, I. Gee (eds.), *Public Health Intelligence*,
DOI 10.1007/978-3-319-28326-5

Printed by Printforce, the Netherlands